PRAISE FOR

You Finished Treatment, Now What?
A Field Guide for Cancer Survivors

"There is an enormous unmet need for relatable, valid, clear, and helpful advice for people after cancer treatment is complete and patients are all too often abandoned to the rocky road of survivorship. Drawing on her own experience as both a practitioner and a patient, Dr Rothenberg ably navigates the world of care and cure with the effortless encouragement of a real pro who really knows and can help you understand what's needed to step into a brighter and better future."

—RICHARD PENSON, MD, MRCP
Associate Professor, Medicine, Harvard Medical School
Clinical Director, Medical Gynecologic Oncology, Medicine, MA General
Hospital

"There is a least common denominator amid the abundance in Dr. Rothenberg's timely, prescient, powerful book: *she understands*. There's more: *she knows what to do* about that whacky penumbral zone just past the cascades of treatment and wobbly assurances that you made it through. The intimate disclosures embedded in her exceptionally rigorous, evidenced framework of clinical savvy and experience, all those doable recommendations, her crisp, substantial ideas for supportive care strategies, all these mean that this book will enduringly touch and engage cancer survivors quickly and uniquely. I've admired this remarkable doctor for many years from my two-decade perch as president of two naturopathic medical institutions. Our faculty, our students, our grads, our profession welcome this book. Her words, chiseled out of the fuss and rattle of so much conversation about surviving and thriving, shifts everything and illuminates the terrain. This book is authentic, accessible, and compassionate. It robustly claims space as the best counsel in the land on this tough issue."

—DAVID J. SCHLEICH, PHD

President Emeritus, National University of Natural Medicine

Cancer Survivor

"In my experience, the last day of anticancer treatment is highly anticipated and is celebrated by many patients. However, at the time of their first follow-up visit, many report that they are surprised that they are feeling anxious and insecure—as if they are waiting for 'the other shoe to drop.' The joy that they had experienced at the completion of treatment had been interrupted by a feeling of being untethered or out of control because they were no longer actively fighting the cancer. These difficult feelings may also be compounded by lingering effects of treatment. This book is a wonderful tool to assist patients in getting through the exciting and challenging post-treatment phase and may help in taking on the role of survivor. Dr. Rothenberg has experienced cancer from 'both sides of the johnny,' and she is able to benefit countless others by sharing her vast knowledge with this book."

—LINDA BORNSTIEN, MD

Former Director, Radiation Oncology, Cooley Dickinson Hospital

"When cancer enters our lives, we look for people who listen, understand, and provide guidance for making wise decisions in this new and unknown land. Reading this book is like sitting down for tea with a friend who's been where you're headed. Dr. Amy Rothenberg has lived what she writes about as a patient, as a family caregiver, and as a medical provider. She knows and respects what different systems of medicine have to offer, and her own life shows that we can weave them together. She is also a wise coach inspiring us to find the unique strengths we can bring to our own health and medical challenges. This is mind-body medicine at its best!"

—ELIZABETH CAHN, PHD

Senior Advisor, Dana-Farber/Harvard Cancer Center Breast Cancer Advocacy Group , Program Director, Cancer Connection, Northampton, MA.

"Personally and professionally, I highly recommend Dr. Amy's book. I have had many family members and friends who have been cancer survivors and thrivers. The quality of their lives was greatly enhanced through the use of nutrition, exercise, meditation, and a myriad of other natural and holistic measures. This book and all of Dr. Rothenberg's approaches create a treatment plan that dovetails and complements conventional cancer care and most importantly encourages physical vitality, mental clarity, and emotional balance—vital for all of us on our healing journeys."

—NANCY HOFREUTER O'HARA, MD, MPH, FAAP

"With massive advancements in cancer treatments, more patients than ever before are entering survivorship. All too often patients are overwhelmed by care when they receive a cancer diagnosis, and just as quickly they may suffer a lack of support during survivorship. Dr. Rothenberg's voice and expertise provide companionship, encouragement, support, and invaluable advice for both patients and practitioners. It is clear that she embodies her advice, and what a privilege it is to have her share her gifts for this population!"

—VEERA MOTASHAW, DO, HMDC
Palliative Care Physician, Cancer Institute,
University of Tennessee Medical Center, Knoxville, TN

"Dr. Rothenberg's grasp of the spectrum of care cancer patients go through is impressive and necessary. She brings the weight and depth of her personal journey as a cancer patient and survivor to the science and spiritual ground of her decades-long practice of natural medicine. Her synthesis and integration of these two areas, often construed as disparate, is nuanced, knowledgeable, intimate, and commanding."

—LINDSAY ROCKWELL, DO
Former Medical Director, Medical Oncology, Massachusetts General Cancer
Center at Cooley Dickinson Hospital, Northampton, MA

"With exquisite sensitivity, Dr. Amy Rothenberg has crafted an excellent book about the most relevant aspects of the healing process from cancer. Inspiring with her own history with cancer, Dr. Rothenberg is a superb guide. She helps sharpen our perception and understanding of the role we play in our own recovery. Cancer does amazing things to our bodies and our emotional beings. It may force us to confront the deeper issues of life and truth. Dr. Rothenberg transforms adversity into promise and possibilities, offering a touch of enlightenment along the way."

—NANCY NOVACK, PHD
Founder of Nancy's List, Cancer Survivor

"Recovering from cancer is not the end of the story, rather the beginning of choices that determine your health for the rest of your life. With humor, solid science, and practical advice, Dr. Rothenberg tells the stories of many patients who followed her advice and regained their vitality. Dr. Rothenberg makes personal her inspirational journey from cancer to robust health."

—JOE PIZZORNO, ND

Co-Author, *Encyclopedia of Natural Medicine*
Founding President, Bastyr University
Chair, Institute for Functional Medicine Board of Directors
Founding Editor of *Integrative Medicine: A Clinician's Journal*

"Early on in the book, Dr. Rothenberg confides how it is 'eye opening to be in the patient chair after so many years as a doctor.' Those words and that firsthand experience are so potent. Though I did it in reverse order—patient with cancer first, later to become a doctor—there is so much resonance in how we met cancer and how we choose to live, experience, and share life. Dr. Rothenberg speaks of empowerment, no matter the outcome, and takes *docere* (Latin, meaning 'teacher') to the next level. And what a great teacher she is—able to articulate a difficult subject with a soothing voice, offering light on what at times is an obscure and darkened path. Thank you for walking with us on this journey and offering a solid set of tools to guide the way."

—NASHA WINTERS, ND, FABNO

Co-Author of *The Metabolic Approach to Cancer* and *Mistletoe and the Emergence of Integrative Oncology*
Co-Founder and Executive Director, Metabolic Terrain Institute of Health

"This book ticks the boxes as both a guide and an inspiration for any person affected by cancer. Dr. Rothenberg has talked the talk, walked the walk, and offers her insight and experience as a licensed naturopathic physician and cancer survivor in a compassionate and useful guide on integrating effective natural medicine approaches. Evidence-informed advice on specific foods, plants, supplements, communication techniques, and more are juxtaposed with personal anecdotes to make this book at once intensely personal and incredibly practical."

—TINA KACZOR, ND, FABNO
Editor in Chief, *The Natural Medicine Journal*
Founding Chair of the Board, Naturopathic Oncology Foundation

"Dr. Rothenberg has created an essential resource for anyone diagnosed with cancer, as well as for everyone involved with that individual, whether a caregiver, a family member, or friend simply wanting to help. With her expertise as a physician, her personal history as a primary caregiver, and as a cancer survivor herself, she thoughtfully provides supportive care strategies for during treatment and for long after. No matter the reader's previous knowledge or level of experience, Dr. Rothenberg guides them to make the changes that can make the difference in addressing these challenging health-care issues. This is a must-read!"

—MARCIA PRENGUBER, ND, FABNO
Former Dean, College of Naturopathic Medicine, University of Bridgeport, CT
Former Director, Integrative Care, Indiana University Heath System,
Center for Cancer Care, Goshen, Indiana
Cancer Survivor

"That Dr. Amy Rothenberg knows her subject is no surprise, given her thirty-six years of clinical practice and as a cancer survivor/thriver herself. It's how she shares her expertise, blending authority, compassion, and humility, that makes *You Finished Treatment, Now What?* a gift. Beautifully written, and full of practical and actionable advice, *You Finished Treatment* belongs in the hands, minds, and hearts of cancer survivors, their families, and clinicians."

—PAUL MITTMAN, ND, EDD
President and CEO, Southwest College of Naturopathic Medicine

"Many books have been published on health and wellness, but Dr. Amy Rothenberg's book *You Finished Treatment, Now What? A Field Guide for Cancer Survivors* is truly the only book on this topic you will need as a patient or practitioner. Dr. Rothenberg's words are full of compassion, intelligence, and most importantly, experience. This book is beyond satisfying in detailing all aspects of what you need to know with regards to cancer survivorship."

—PINA LOGIUDICE, ND, LAC
Author of *The Little Book of Healthy Beauty—
Simple Daily Habits to Get You Glowing*
Founder, Innersource Health, New York City, Frequent Guest on *Dr. Oz*

"The public realizes that 'long Covid' is an actual diagnosis. It's useful to apply the same concept to those who complete cancer care. Your cancer might be kept at bay for years. Or in the case of my own tonsillar cancer, it may be successfully treated, but the radiation and chemotherapy create shifting, lifelong challenges. In either case, it could be described as 'long cancer.' Among the many values of Dr. Rothenberg's book to the cancer thriver, literature is one core to her profession. She always works with the unique individual toward the goal of optimal health as the patient frames it. It helps that Dr. Rothenberg has extraordinary skill with both the written and spoken word, and has abiding concern for each individual she meets and treats, which also comes through in her prose."

—JOHN WEEKS
Former Editor in Chief, *The Journal of Alternative and Complementary Medicine*
Publisher and Editor, *Integrator Blog News & Reports*

"Dr. Rothenberg's compendium for cancer survivors and thrivers presents a rejuvenative and restorative strategy for those entering the post-treatment phase, a strategy often missing in the current medical paradigm. It also offers a pathway toward improving 'healthspan,' or the time one thrives in health. This is a comprehensive book in its coverage of diet, nutrition, exercise, sleep, mental health, and the palette of integrative possibilities available to all of us who seek healthy, fulfilling lives."

—RENÉE ROSSI, MD, MFA, MA-AY

"Dr. Amy Rothenberg has written a heartfelt, informed, and action-oriented primer for those who have finished cancer treatment. Speaking from personal experience and as a practicing naturopathic doctor for over thirty-six years, Dr. Rothenberg is an ideal guide for those folks asking, 'Now what?' post cancer treatment. Sharing specific knowledge about how our bodies work and how we can strengthen ourselves is timely, not only for cancer survivors but really for anyone interested in bettering their health and vitality! Share this book with your loved ones."

—MICHELLE SIMON, PHD, ND
President and CEO, Institute for Natural Medicine

"Dr. Rothenberg is a practitioner whom I have admired for a very long time. So, I am not surprised that she is filling the gap in conventional cancer care. In this book, Dr. Rothenberg is empowering cancer survivors with an answer to the question 'What now?' In my experience as an integrative specialist for cancer patients, the biggest misstep in conventional treatment is that patients are without direction as to what interventions to make and keep for the long term. I am so happy Dr. Rothenberg stepped up when she saw the need to educate those who need it most."

—CHRISTIAN GONZALEZ, ND
Integrative Oncology, Chronic Disease and General Medicine

"As a cancer survivor and trauma therapist having to navigate surgery and radiation, I could not have done it as successfully without the expertise, wisdom, and compassionate guidance of Dr. Rothenberg. Her unusual wisdom and ability create a breakthrough book for survivors to navigate life after traditional cancer treatment. These recommendations mitigate the oftentimes long-lasting, physically and emotionally disruptive symptoms. Dr. Rothenberg's natural approach provided me a road map to help strengthen my immune system, have more confidence in my recovery, and restore my overall health. Her book is critically important and provides a compassionate and knowledgeable support system for cancer patients and survivors!"

—DR. ALAN GOLDBERG
Sports Performance Consultant
Competitivedge.com
Cancer Survivor

"As a therapist, this book gives me tools to help my clients who are cancer survivors/thrivers. My wish is that every oncology department gives this book to patients as they complete treatment. Dr. Rothenberg's book is a holistic empowerment guide on all aspects of 'what's next' after cancer care ends. It helps people move beyond being traumatized by cancer to being empowered by their self-care. Dr Rothenberg gives hope."

—ANGE DIBENEDETTO, EDD, SEP

Trauma Specialist Psychotherapist

"Dr Rothenberg relies on her own experience as both patient and medical practitioner to provide not just hope but evidenced approaches to support an integrated medical model. Adopting the interventions she shares changes the terrain within each individual, providing healthful resiliency. Sharing the teachings of her joyful stories as well as serving as a comprehensive guide for effecting real change in our medical approach to cancer, this book is both long overdue and timely."

—JULIANNE M. FORBES, MBA, ND

"Dr Amy Rothenberg offers her loving hand and compassionate heart in masterfully guiding survivors. This book is a breath of ocean air, a rare gem, and a must-have for any cancer patient who is searching for multifaceted guidance and support into the holistic world of self-care and natural medicine after treatment. She has walked hospital oncology halls and has creatively and generously offered her thirty-six years of wisdom as a naturopathic physician and teacher. Her delightful sense of humor and tenderheartedness is apparent on every page. This book is her gift to us and a true treasure for anyone's library."

—LINDA LEVINE, DC

"A must-have resource for anyone who feels that they need more answers to proactively support themselves after cancer treatment. With this book, Dr. Rothenberg delivers clear and actionable solutions that comprehensively answer the question 'Now what?' Offering a unique, hard-earned perspective that blends her lived experience as a patient navigating cancer care with her decades of practice as a naturopathic physician, this book can save you hours of research, and empower you with the hope that vibrant health is possible with the right knowledge."

—ROB KACHKO ND, LIC AC

President, The American Association of Naturopathic Physicians 2019–2021

"When an oncologist reported I had stage 4 aggressive double hit B-cell lymphoma, my approach was for the doctors to take care of the treatment and for me to focus on supporting myself through the treatment. Dr. Rothenberg provided the guidance I needed during a very confusing and frightening time. As a cancer survivor in remission, her prescriptions are an integral part of my life. Her depth of knowledge, personal experience, and authenticity is a gift I shall be ever grateful for. She has documented all this in a book for others as an indispensable resource for cancer survivors and their families."

—SANDRA WYNER ANDREW

Montessori Educational Consultant

"In *You Finished Treatment, Now What?* Dr. Rothenberg offers up unparalleled wisdom, expertise, and advice for cancer survivors. As the wife of one of her patients and the sister of another, both cancer survivors thriving under her care, I can testify to the power of these approaches. Dr. Rothenberg's simple, clear, proven, and powerful recommendations for physical, emotional, and cognitive health are an essential complement to the protocols your oncologists prescribe. As a bonus, caregivers also benefit from Dr Rothenberg's exercise, nutrition, and lifestyle recommendations. I feel better than I have in years. Read this book to thrive, long after your cancer treatments end."

—SARA SCHLEY, MBA
Founder and CEO, Seed Systems

"I was on a roll. Three continents and four countries a week. In the US alone, three medical practices: NY, Chicago, and San Francisco. Production crews, TV programs, radio shows in multiple countries. In Ecuador I was chair of osteopathic medicine and chief science officer for the first osteopathic medical hospital in the country. Then I hit a wall. It was shattering. Four death experiences, five surgeries, with severe anesthesia and medication reactions. I was bedridden for two years, a prisoner in my own body. But the winds of resurrection blow from a place of death and rebirth. Dr. Rothenberg's book is that wind. It's a road map, a way back. Sooner or later someone in your family is going to face cancer and need this book. *You Finished Treatment, Now What?* is a must-read."

—DANE SHEPHERD DO
Osteopathic Physician and Surgeon

You Finished Treatment, Now What?
A Field Guide for Cancer Survivors
by Dr. Amy Rothenberg

ISBN 978-1-64663-793-5

Published by

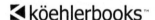 köehlerbooks™

3705 Shore Drive
Virginia Beach, VA 23455
800-435-4811
www.koehlerbooks.com

YOU FINISHED TREATMENT, NOW WHAT?

A Field Guide for Cancer Survivors

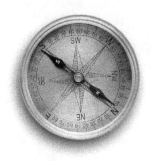

DR. AMY ROTHENBERG

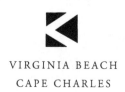

VIRGINIA BEACH
CAPE CHARLES

To Joan Lois Rothenberg, beloved daughter, sister, cousin, aunt, and friend, who put up the good fight many more times than most, who taught us to be in the moment, and who faced adversity with humor and grace. Rest in peace, dear sister.

Disclaimer

THE INFORMATION PROVIDED in this book is not meant to diagnose or treat any medical condition. For diagnosis or treatment of any health problem, consult your medical provider. References are offered for informational purposes only and do not constitute endorsement of any website or other source. Readers should be aware that websites and reference links listed in this book may change. Science and medicine are constantly evolving. New research and clinical experience will lead to changes in recommendations. The author, editors, publisher, and any other party involved in this work encourage readers to verify the information contained in these pages, and to consult with regulated health-care providers for specific, individualized recommendations.

Table of Contents

Introduction

YOU'D THINK THE last day of chemo or the final radiation treatment would be a time to rejoice and celebrate. But for many cancer patients, the last day of treatment is soon followed by a sense of dread and despair. The fighting stance and the rallying cries end. The outpouring of support slows. It's on to "life as usual," which is not easy if you don't feel well, and medical "active surveillance" seems to be served up with a hefty portion of stress and anxiety.

I know this terrain intimately, as a cancer survivor/thriver and as a licensed naturopathic doctor. I was living a healthy lifestyle and blessed with pristine health when diagnosed with breast and then ovarian cancer in 2014. I wrote[1] extensively on the topic of using natural medicine *during* my own cancer treatment. It was certainly eye-opening to be in the patient chair after so many years as a doctor.

I had the great fortune of receiving state-of-the-art conventional treatment at a world-renowned teaching hospital, and locally in my smaller, hometown cancer center. I was in excellent hands with some of the smartest people I have ever met. I also had guidance and encouragement from brilliant colleagues in the naturopathic profession who specialize in integrative oncology.

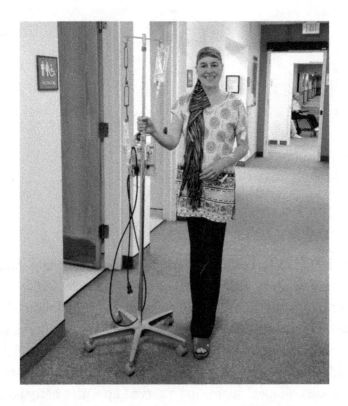

Dr. Rothenberg at her last chemotherapy appointment, 2014

Integrative oncology is defined as a "patient-centered, evidence-informed field of comprehensive cancer care that uses mind-body practices, natural products, and lifestyle modifications from different traditions alongside conventional cancer treatments. It prioritizes safety and best available evidence to offer appropriate therapeutic interventions along with conventional care."[2] I believe that as patient demand and research continue to grow, integrative oncology will be the standard of care for every patient going through cancer care and throughout their survivorship years.

I have been lucky over my career to have warm and meaningful relationships with colleagues. We consult with each other on difficult cases and share information. Because no doctor should treat themselves, when I was diagnosed I immediately reached out to a number of naturopathic doctors, who were enormously generous and caring, for which I am eternally grateful. My goals with naturopathic approaches were several: to enhance efficacy of my conventional care, prevent or minimize side effects, address side effects that arose, and to glean general support throughout my time of treatment.

My naturopathic physician providers regularly scour the medical research, distill complicated biochemistry related to cancer and its treatment, and provide up-to-date information *after* my care as well. During that entire time and since, I've also had unparalleled "in-house" help from my devoted husband and partner, Paul Herscu, ND, MPH, a veritable research phenom who left no stone unturned to find the best medical paths forward, seamlessly blending my conventional and natural medicine plans, while at the same time offering endless encouragement and comfort.

After cancer treatment, I have committed to many of the approaches described in this book and continue to take my health, and my ability to impact my health, seriously. I kicked up my already healthy relationship with exercise, I further tidied up my diet, I let go of certain commitments and people in my life that caused undue stress, I added specific anticancer supplements to my daily intake, and so much more.

I continue to work with my naturopathic physician colleagues as well as my oncologists. We create a treatment plan that dovetails with the details of my medical story and also takes into account my temperament and my capacity to do the work that is part of getting well and staying healthy. I continue, years out, with approaches that encourage physical vitality, spiritual peace, mental clarity, and emotional balance, while doing all I can to reduce my risk of recurrence.

Should my cancer ever return, which I deeply hope it does not, I will always feel I did as much as I possibly could to protect the life I hold so dear. Creating a plan, committing to it, and modifying as needed is empowering. I aim to model much of the content of this book for my patients, understanding firsthand what it means to be disciplined without becoming rigid, what it takes to make changes without disrupting my family life, and how to make small sacrifices while also taking pleasure in the day-to-day moments of my life.

My perspective is further defined by cancer patients and survivors I've treated in my practice over the last thirty-six years. I offer evidence-based information alongside a cheerleading nature. I emphasize lifestyle medicine: how you eat, exercise, reduce stress, decrease exposure to environmental toxins, and more. I employ a full toolbox of natural medicines to help address specific health challenges. I remind patients it's possible to shift modifiable risk factors that may have led you to be more susceptible to developing cancer in the first place. As a most central mission, I want you to have good quality of life—the capacity to enjoy yourself, do the work or play you want, and connect with the important people in your life in meaningful ways.

I work collaboratively with patients' skilled conventional medical providers. And as proof of natural and lifestyle-medicine emerges, I see more and more interest in and respect for such approaches from medical colleagues. An integrative approach is always ideal, taking the best from all parts of medicine. No two patient stories are the same, but some elements ring true: we all need information, creative problem-solving, and compassion as we navigate post-treatment life.

And the need is ever expanding. The number of survivors is growing[3] as treatment for all kinds of cancer improves. By the 2040s, the US will be home to more than twenty-six million cancer survivors. In addition, there will be many other people living productive lives *with* cancer while taking medications and using other approaches that help keep them alive. Improvements in the world of oncology are made all the time, and many of us are recipients of those advances.

Nonetheless, there is a time I call "mopping up," where we work to reverse collateral damage from cancer treatment. Research[4] shows that cancer survivors often report physical and psychological challenges well after cancer care has ended and that their needs often go unmet. You may struggle with lingering side effects of treatment. Long-term side effects may begin during active cancer care and continue after care ends. Challenges vary dramatically based on your treatment type, length of treatment, other health concerns, underlying genetics, and lifestyle choices.

Common side effects include low blood counts, lymphedema, "chemo brain," skin issues, weight loss, weight gain, peripheral neuropathy, digestive disturbances, anxiety, depression, insomnia, and fatigue. That said, in my decades of practice, I've seen cancer survivors with symptoms involving nearly every system of the body, including far-reaching cognitive and emotional issues. Of course, some survivors may have had these concerns *before* being diagnosed and treated for cancer. But for others, these symptoms are entirely new and most unwelcome— like another bad chapter layered over an already overwhelming ordeal of a cancer diagnosis and treatment.

You may have had no symptoms or only mild symptoms at the time of diagnosis. Perhaps you had a few risk factors and previously enjoyed good health. Being diagnosed with cancer may have been especially shocking. Then, as symptoms arose from conventional treatments, which by design can be harsh in order to get the job done, it may have felt like a further blow. This book can help you right the ship, to unwind from some of the trauma and impact of life-saving conventional care.

Health-care providers of all types will see a plethora of cancer survivors through various phases of life, yet provider advice that is proactive regarding lifestyle and natural medicine is lagging, even while the scientific research has made and continues to make great strides.

I write this book to fill the gap of information and offer guidance for survivors, to help you rebuild and restore, and to support the innate resilience of the human body and spirit. And for people living with cancer, in and out of treatment, many for years to come, you'll also find actionable ideas. Perhaps you have a genetic propensity for cancer or have another illness, the treatment for which puts you at risk for cancer. Study these guidelines. Family members and caregivers may benefit from reading these pages. And I write these chapters for medical providers, in hopes that more of you will offer or at least endorse such recommendations, or refer patients to a practitioner who has pertinent expertise.

Some offerings are general, others more pointed toward specific complaints. I share information and experience to encourage you to be proactive about your health instead of waiting around for cancer to develop or return. I am also interested in helping you address the psycho-emotional element of your story, because for most everyone, psychological symptoms impact the way we move through life, in sickness *and* in health. Emotions influence the physical body in predictable and important-to-understand ways.

The internet is overflowing with information and testimonials; some may be helpful, some may do nothing at all, and of course, some may be harmful. This book helps orient you to better navigate the field of integrative oncology.

You do not need to take up every suggestion written in this book, even if research and clinical experience from each section show promise or results. No one can do everything that could potentially be cancer preventive. There is simply not enough time in the day. Some patients drive themselves—and their loved ones—a bit weary trying to do all that is possible, at great expenditure of time, resources, and energy. Remember, your body reflects the habitual, not the occasional. Certain approaches will have more appeal than others depending on your personality, temperament, time, resources, support, and other factors.

Being kind and gentle with yourself is another essential component of healing. I prefer when my patients make slow, gradual, more permanent changes, instead of trying to change everything all at once. If you already live a healthy lifestyle, you may find some ways to amplify your efforts, or you may discover ways to fine-tune with natural medicines aimed to address particular residual complaints.

Before you embark on creating a plan for yourself, consider working with a licensed naturopathic doctor or other medical provider well versed in this material as part of your medical dream team. As with all good medicine, specific treatment plans need to be individualized to the patient. If you came to me or to a colleague, we'd want to know what type of cancer you had, where it was, what approaches were taken, and which—if any— side effects you've experienced. We'd want to know about current or residual health issues from treatment. From there we'd map out a strategy and a plan.

In addition to using the information in these pages, please keep up your medical oversight, including patient visits, laboratory analysis, and pertinent scanning. This remains essential, as early discovery of either new cancers or metastatic illness is always best. A number of organizations regularly update recommendations for follow-up care based on types of cancers. I support this kind of surveillance entirely.

I write this book about being a doctor, being a patient, getting sick, getting better, and staying healthy, and how it is possible— to one degree or another—for you and so many other cancer survivors. I am dedicated to helping you improve your capacity for regaining and maintaining your health, and for best possible health outcomes. Natural medicine cannot help every person or every complaint, but I feel sad when I hear patients say, "Well, I'm lucky to be alive. I can live with this." Let's face it: we're all lucky to be alive. *And* quality of life matters.

I want to help without giving false hope. I wish you the clarity of mind to take up appropriate approaches, the discipline needed to stay the course, and resilience to handle setbacks or challenges. Knowledge about your body, biochemistry, and physiology can help inform your decision-making related to both lifestyle and treatment approaches. Knowledge is power. Take this information and make it your own.

With wishes for your good health and vitality,

Amy Rothenberg ND
Amherst, Massachusetts
March 14, 2022

How to Use this Book

ALTHOUGH I WOULD like you to read this book in its entirety, I know that all sorts of demands compete for your time! I suggest you first read the parts of this book that interest you most, with an understanding that whole-person, whole-medicine approaches will have the most benefit. Over time, you can go back and fill in the chapters you skipped over. Each section is freestanding, so while it's intended to be appreciated in context with the other chapters, adoption of *any* of the recommendations described or lifestyle modifications offered will also be helpful. Incremental and enduring changes are best—not a total overhaul that is often unsustainable. In chapter 17, you will find more specific advice for common complaints experienced after cancer treatment.

Please note that I do not include suggested dosages in my recommendations for nutritional supplements or botanical medicines. This is because you have your unique health history and current set of complaints and underlying physical tendencies. A good amount of one herbal medicine for you may be too much for another person. This is less of a *how-to* book and more of a *how-to-think* book, about general and specific ideas related to after-cancer complaints, and also about how to create an internal environment less hospitable to the return of cancer.

Another way to use this book is to share this information with your health-care providers. Use ideas and references as a place to start a conversation and ask your questions. Personally, I love an informed, knowledgeable patient and welcome the opportunity to learn from them. Not every doctor feels that way, it's true, but having a resource to reference will hopefully help support those conversations.

Lastly, I hope that using this book and leaning into its recommendations will help you realize that you're in very good company, that there are literally thousands of other cancer survivors/thrivers working hard to regain and maintain health. Because this number is constantly growing and there is more interest in natural medicine approaches than ever before, research is galloping and of great interest to many of us. As our understanding of human physiology and cancer biology evolves, may we all be the recipients of both advances in conventional cancer care and newfound understanding of how lifestyle and natural medicine approaches improve quality of life and health outcomes.

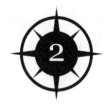

How to Talk So Your Oncologist Listens, and Listen So Your Oncologist Talks*

WHEN YOU ARE pursuing natural, integrative medicine alongside or after conventional care, you may have information to share with your oncologist and certainly questions to ask. A vast majority of cancer patients are doing, using, or practicing some form of integrative medicine during and after conventional cancer care. Learning the best ways for you to communicate, share information, and ask questions is important. Having self-agency, feeling empowered, and maintaining positive interactions with providers are all part of the healing process.

The oncology profession has spent time examining[5] patient–practitioner communication and continues to research what approaches work best. You and many other patients may struggle to grasp all the science and medical-ese behind a cancer diagnosis and treatment plan, or post-care testing and treatment, especially when feeling stressed in the clinical or hospital setting and with information flying faster than you can absorb. The use of online patient portals has made information sharing easier[6] but sometimes all the more overwhelming. This is true for those in treatment, those who have completed conventional care, and those living with cancer.

Here are some guidelines to help support you in effective communications as you navigate being a survivor/thriver and to help you gain the most from your doctor visits with the least amount of stress.

✦   **BRING A FRIEND OR SUPPORT PERSON TO ALL YOUR APPOINTMENTS.** You don't have to go it alone. If you do not have anyone to bring, ask if a social worker or patient advocate can accompany you on your visits. Many oncology facilities have people on staff for just this purpose. Enlisting a support person might take a little more time and some scheduling coordination, but it is worth the effort.

✦   **CREATE A FOLDER OR NOTEBOOK** or place on your computer where you keep and organize all relevant information. Date everything collected. Create categories for easy access, such as pathology reports, laboratory results, the chemotherapy prescribed, radiation treatment schedule, surgical notes, genetic testing, natural medicine recommendations, insurance information, and so on.

✦   **CREATE AN UP-TO-DATE "HISTORY OF PRESENT ILLNESS SUMMARY,"** a one-to-two page synopsis of your cancer-related story—to share with any new provider and to refer to during an initial visit. Delineate date of diagnosis, what the diagnosis was, if you had a biopsy, what it revealed, what treatments you took or are currently taking, and how you tolerated or tolerate those treatments. Include your main *current* symptoms or concerns. Write down any over-the-counter or natural medicine approaches you have tried or currently use as well as any drugs you take.

◆ **PRINT OUT OR HAVE HANDY RECENT LAB WORK AND SCAN REPORTS,** as relevant, unless your new provider can easily access on the clinic or hospital portal. You may want to review these pages, especially before meeting with a new provider, and update periodically. The more information you can share, the more informed conversation you will have.

◆ **BRING YOUR OWN HEALTHY FOOD OR SNACKS TO HOSPITALS OR CLINICS WHEN POSSIBLE.** I often have a good chuckle when I observe the processed, high trans-fats snacks and sugary drinks set out for free at many cancer centers. There might as well be a sign nearby that reads, *Eat this and you can be a repeat customer!* Bring your own water bottle and stay hydrated. Learn where the bathrooms are at the clinic.

◆ **REMEMBER, YOU WILL OFTEN ENCOUNTER LONG WAITS.** Bring a book, tablet, phone, knitting, or whatever you like for entertainment or distraction. Try not to become upset about waiting. Reframe it in your mind as welcome quiet time where you can practice your breathing exercises, do a crossword puzzle, listen to music, or whatever you please. If your provider typically runs thirty to forty-five minutes late, working with other patients, perhaps they will also take extra time with you should you ever need it. Some clinics allow you to check in and then will send a text when your doctor is ready for you. I take advantage of this by going for long walks around the hospital or grounds, which helps me clear my head, move my body, and relax. During one visit where my provider was over an hour late, I logged in 5,000 steps up and around the various floors and hallways of the hospital!

✦ **CONSIDER MEETING YOUR PROVIDERS FULLY DRESSED**—as a way to be a person in their eyes first, a patient second. As a doctor, if I need to do a complete or relevant physical exam, I will leave the room to offer the patient privacy for changing into a gown after having met them.

✦ **DO YOUR HOMEWORK, OR HAVE A LOVED ONE DO IT FOR YOU.** Read about options related to your after-treatment care. Are there any new approaches being offered for people with a similar diagnosis once treatment is complete? You can ask, "What can we *actively do* to prevent recurrence?" I am not satisfied with simply testing and ramping up surveillance. There are so many other powerful approaches: you can help support immune function; get the mind working on your behalf; use nutrition to optimize recovery, strength, and energy; employ botanical medicine to help with sleep or anxiety or constipation. The list goes on. There are also whole-person medicines to help prevent and address other acute illnesses that arise. There are ways to create an internal environment less hospitable to cancer. These are the very subjects of this book.

✦ **CONSIDER ASKING FOR A REFERRAL** to the person at your medical facility overseeing clinical trials. Often there are relevant trials you might be eligible for and interested in. Even if you are not eligible or interested in a clinical trial currently available, it is wise to establish this relationship, because you may need to circle back around to that department or individual one day.

✦ **KNOW THAT THERE IS A WHOLE WORLD OF TRANSLATIONAL MEDICINE,**[7] described as "a rapidly growing discipline in biomedical research that aims to expedite the discovery of new diagnostic tools and treatments by using a multidisciplinary, highly collaborative, 'bench-to-bedside' approach." In other words, there is information generated by researchers that—due to regulatory concerns, financial stake of scientists and inventors, governmental red tape, and more—are not immediately available to patients in need. The scientific community is getting better here, but we have a long way to go. This is a much-needed step, as many well-researched, evidence-based, effective treatments exist that have simply not made it to the clinic yet.

✦ **BRING EVIDENCE FOR THE EFFICACY OF APPROACHES YOU ARE CONSIDERING OR USING** when visiting a health provider. One tool you can use is Pubmed, an online clearing house for much medical and scientific research, maintained by the National Center of Biotechnology Information, part of the National Library of Medicine. If you understand that the herb *Curcumin longa* might help reduce inflammation and prevent cancer recurrence, for example, but your oncologist is raising an eyebrow, you can go to your search engine and type in these three words: *Pubmed, curcumin, cancer.* Many articles will come up.[8] If you don't have much of a science background, many of the articles on Pubmed will be challenging to wade through, but you can read the summary and get the gist. Bring hard copies with you to share, and ask your doctor's opinion. Another resource is the Oncology Association of Naturopathic Physicians website,[9] which has sections on all aspects of oncology research related to natural and integrative medicine. You can also find relevant research by checking the endnotes in this book, as I include references for most all items or strategies discussed.

✦ **HAVE YOUR WRITTEN LIST OF QUESTIONS AND CONCERNS** with you and be sure to let your doctor know from the outset that you have a number of questions to ask. Then, make sure to write down the answers or have the person with you do so. When I was in treatment, I was often too worried or too tired to take in much of what happened at my frequent doctor visits. That's why I always brought a support person with me to remind me to ask questions, to write answers, and for general support. Some months after my care ended, I knew I was doing better when I told my husband, "It's okay, honey. I can go by myself."

✦ **THESE SAME SUGGESTIONS APPLY FOR THOSE LIVING WITH CANCER** who continue to have follow-up visits. You are often seeing providers who are experts in their fields, with jam-packed schedules. You want to make the best use of your time and theirs, and to leave, when possible, with actionable information.

✦ **CONSIDER ASKING YOUR PROVIDER IF YOU CAN MAKE AN AUDIO RECORDING OF YOUR VISIT.** Many of my patients ask, and I am happy to oblige. Some but not all providers will agree to let you record; there may be concerns with liability or words taken out of context, so please ask ahead of time. Everyone learns and remembers information differently. It's amazing to listen to a recording later and learn what you may have missed the first time around. Advocate for communication approaches that are effective for you.

✦ **ASK WHAT THE BEST WAY TO CONTACT YOUR DOCTOR IS.** Some providers are happy to field emails, while others discourage this or do not provide email information. I urge my patients to obtain direct numbers or emails to reach the doctor or, more commonly, their support staff, as well as for laboratory or diagnostic imaging centers. This way, appointments can be made easily, and questions or concerns can be registered in a timely fashion, without long waits or the maze of automated telephone directories.

✦ **LEARN TO USE THE ONLINE PORTALS** most clinics and hospitals now offer. Create a username and password and keep those somewhere you will remember. Consider sharing login information with a trusted family member if desired. Many portals have areas for making or changing appointments, viewing and paying bills, sending a brief note or question to your provider, reviewing records of your procedures, treatment, and laboratory results, and accessing other support services.

I have personally found the online portals useful, timely, and helpful—once I figured out how to navigate them! That said, with all that easy access, you might feel overwhelmed with *too much* information. Don't feel you need to examine every piece of your health history, laboratory results, or scan reports all the time. Access the portal as needed. Or deputize someone else to look for you if it causes undo stress.

After one set of follow-up scans to my chest, pelvis, and abdomen, I got the thumbs-up from my provider once the results were in. That all-clear message is always joyous. My oncologist, then speaking doctor to doctor, sat me down and pulled my images up on the screen, and proceeded to show me body part after body part where I had no evidence of disease. I found it overwhelming. About halfway through this generous anatomy exercise, I said, "You know what, I'm good with the simple *all clear*," which my loving doctor heard loud and clear, and never offered that kind of exhaustive review again.

✦ **RECALL THE SECOND OPINION.** Patients diagnosed with cancer are entitled to a second opinion, and it's never too late to ask for one. Even when care is completed, if you are looking for other approaches to help improve your health or hopefully reduce your risk for recurrence, another conventional oncologist may have a fresh perspective. And while we should all foremost be interested in the person who has the correct technical skills to match our specific complaint, bedside manner counts. You have the right to change providers if you need someone different, though there are definite benefits to working with same person or people over time. Hopefully they will learn about you as a person, recall the details of your story, and provide direct information, alongside support and encouragement.

I had one primary-care provider who kept asking me on annual visits if I'd had my annual mammogram. Since I'd had both breasts removed years earlier and no longer needed mammograms, the fact that she either did not recall or did not take time to review my chart before seeing me wore thin. I eventually changed my primary-care physician to someone who sees me as a unique individual and recalls at least some very basic parts of my health history.

✦ **EXPRESS GRATITUDE AND KINDNESS TO YOUR PROVIDERS.** Thank-you notes, small tokens of appreciation, and kind words go a long way in conveying your appreciation. Who does not want to be appreciated and reminded of the positive impact of their work?

Every year when I complete a summertime triathlon, I send a picture of myself at the finish line with a short note thanking all the *many* providers and other support people who helped me during the time I was in treatment and who continue to look after me. I hope they feel my enduring gratitude! If possible, aim to be *that* patient everyone enjoys. Try to remember or write down names of staff, nurses, phlebotomists, and administrative staff, bring small offerings, and lean in when you can. When you write thank-you notes, be specific!

✦ **IF YOU FEEL POWERLESS AND OVERWHELMED, TRY TO CREATE AN ISLAND OF PERSONAL POWER AND SPACE** and ownership in your life and in your medical and healing efforts. I try to help my patients with this. For example, when I make naturopathic recommendations and have more than one way to accomplish the same goals, I like to offer choices. Once I understand your values and goals and we discuss options, we can have a shared decision-making process. When your provider makes a recommendation, you can ask if there are other options you should know about. Shared decision-making in medicine has been studied[10] and found to have a positive impact on both patients and doctors.

✦ **IF YOU HEAR SOMETHING, SAY SOMETHING.** At follow-up visits with your oncology team, remember that you're allowed to question your doctor; you're entitled to understand everything that might take place or be recommended. Doctors need feedback too, but cancer survivors often feel somewhere between utter thankfulness for being alive and paralyzing fear of recurrence. No need to be overly demanding or pesky, but keep asking your questions, and keep pushing for answers.

✦ **HALT UNWANTED COMMENTS, STORIES, AND ADVICE** from coworkers, friends, and relatives. Perhaps because of the internet or the number of people touched by cancer, *everyone* has ideas and recommendations. Everyone's an "expert." I personally found it exhausting to have to listen to advice I was not going to take—and sometimes, any advice at all.

Another experience many cancer patients and survivors share with me is that you can become a magnet for everyone else's cancer stories—just about the last thing in the world most of us want to hear. I found it very helpful to come up with some pat responses and use clear, strong language, as in "Oh, let me stop you there! I am not taking any advice, but thanks so much for your concern." Or one hand up: "NO cancer stories—I MEAN IT!" Or a precomposed email ready to send: *I am confident with the team I have put together and the plan we have created. Thank you for your concern and thoughts, but I won't be responding further to this email! Sincerely, xxx.*

A particular non-favorite of mine are people I see infrequently who somehow put a "cancer" tag on me, so whenever they see me, they ask in an overly sweet voice, leaning in with what I am sure is sincere concern, "Oh, how are *you*?" This bothers me because I am, thankfully, fine, living a wonderful and full life where cancer is no longer my main focus. But even if that were not the case, I resent being pulled back into the cancer world by another person who really has no idea. My general response is "I'm fantastic, just did a triathlon last month. How are *you*?" No one wants to be put in a box, especially not a box that has a big *CANCER* label written on it. In my clinic, I may role-play with my patients so they get the hang of speaking their minds—being courteous enough, appreciating others' concerns, but being clear about defined needs and preferences.

✦ **HERE'S WHAT I'D LIKE TO EMPHASIZE:** With your conventional care team and hopefully input from a licensed naturopathic doctor or integrative-medicine provider, you can create the best possible plan going forward. Then you're going to grab onto the plan and commit to it. From the world of scuba diving we have the following mantra: *We're going to plan the dive and dive the plan*—and not second-guess our decisions. It's the same for cancer survivors/thrivers. We may need to *modify* approaches, and we'll welcome new information for consideration or integration, but we are going to be confident in our plan, moving forward without regrets.

Communication is at the heart of healing, so optimizing your capacity to both share and take in information from your oncologist, while finding your own voice and strength in the process, is an essential part of going through cancer treatment. And it is important whether therapies are stopped, completed, or ongoing.

*Chapter title adapted from *How to Talk So Your Kids Listen and Listen So Your Kids Talk* by Farber and Mazlich, a wonderful best-selling book, and my own personal parenting bible.[11]

Naturopathic Medicine Explained

I LOVE MY profession and was blessed to find it early in my life. I have written extensively about the philosophy, education, and training of naturopathic doctors as well as my own journey to becoming a naturopathic doctor elsewhere[12] but will review some of the basics here.

Naturopathic medicine is a distinct system of medicine that skillfully combines historic therapeutic traditions with modern science to restore and optimize health. Naturopathic doctors gather information from patients using the patient intake and physical exam as well as pertinent laboratory and imaging investigation, alongside understanding a patient's lifestyle, environmental stressors, and health goals.

Naturopathic doctors (NDs) are educated and trained at accredited naturopathic medical colleges. Naturopathic doctors articulate and consistently apply the Therapeutic Order[13] to delineate the natural sequence in which care should be recommended, in order to provide the greatest benefit to the patient with the least potential for side effects.

The Therapeutic Order

1. **REMOVE OBSTACLES TO HEALTH.** The first step in returning to health is to remove the entities that disturb health, such as poor diet, digestive disturbances, and chronic or excessive stress levels. NDs create patient plans based on an individual's obstacles to health in order to change and improve the terrain in which an illness develops. This allows additional, more pointed therapeutics to have the most beneficial impact.

2. **STIMULATE SELF-HEALING MECHANISMS.** NDs use therapies to stimulate and strengthen the body's innate self-healing and curative capacity. These therapies include modalities such as clinical nutrition, botanical medicine, hydrotherapy, homeopathy, acupuncture, lifestyle interventions, the exercise prescription, hands-on approaches, nutritional supplements, and counseling.

3. **STRENGTHEN WEAKENED SYSTEMS.** Systems that need repair are addressed by applying approaches from a full toolbag of therapeutics that enhance specific tissues, organs, or systems, including those listed above.

4. **CORRECT STRUCTURAL INTEGRITY.** Physical modalities such as spinal manipulation, massage therapy, osteopathic manipulation, craniosacral therapy, and others are used to improve and maintain skeletal and musculature integrity, which in turn help with circulation, mobility, digestion, and more.

5. **USE NATURAL SUBSTANCES TO RESTORE AND REGENERATE.** Naturopathic medicine's primary objective is to restore health, not to treat pathology. However, when a specific pathology must be addressed, NDs prioritize safe, effective, natural substances that do not add toxicity or additionally burden an already distressed system.

6. **USE PHARMACOLOGIC SUBSTANCES TO HALT PROGRESSIVE PATHOLOGY.** There is a time and place for drugs, and NDs are trained in pharmacology and how to use pharmaceutical drugs when necessary. NDs prescribe these agents, or if state laws do not allow, NDs refer to medical colleagues. The scope of practice and pharmacy prescriptions are governed by state naturopathic licensing boards and vary from state to state at the time of this book's publication.

7. **USE HIGH-FORCE, INVASIVE MODALITIES.** These include surgery, radiation, and chemotherapy. When life, limb, or function must be preserved, NDs refer patients to MD/DO colleagues who are expert in these areas. At the same time, NDs use complementary or supportive therapies to enhance efficacy, decrease side effects, address side effects that arise, and to help support resilience when treatments are completed.

Naturopathic doctors receive training in the same biomedical and diagnostic sciences as medical doctors and osteopathic doctors (DOs). Naturopathic medical education curricula include certain areas of study not covered in conventional medical school. The result is a comprehensive, rigorous, and well-rounded scientific medical education that is both comparable and complementary to that of MDs and DOs. For more information on how naturopathic doctors are educated, trained, and licensed, and to find a licensed naturopathic doctor, see the American Association of Naturopathic Physicians' comprehensive website: https://naturopathic.org.

While naturopathic doctors are trained in primary care,[14] like conventional medical doctors, some NDs specialize. Naturopathic specialty associations exist for endocrinology, environmental medicine, gastroenterology, parenteral therapies, pediatrics, primary care physicians, psychiatry, homeopathy, and oncology.

Naturopathic doctors have extensive training in behavioral medicine, which helps empowering patients to make and sustain lifestyle changes that improve health. We work to help patients understand and address the underlying social, emotional, and psychological patterns that influence their health. NDs use a broad range of therapies applied according to philosophical underpinnings as described above.

NDs work to support your body's innate capacity to heal. We aim to treat you as a whole person with an individualized treatment plan. NDs prioritize and value the "doctor as teacher" concept and aim to work collaboratively in a way that empowers you in your own medical care. This general description of the profession applies beautifully to cancer survivors, as described in the rest of this volume. NDs are also trained to work collaboratively with providers across the medical landscape. Increasingly, NDs work in integrative medical centers as valued team members.

The Oncology Association of Naturopathic Physicians (OncANP) specialty organization is a robust group of providers and students who focus on treating those whose lives have been touched by cancer. The OncANP published its "Principles of Care,"[15] which is available to the general public. It describes the ways NDs work with cancer patients in the context of the broader oncology world. The hallmarks of these principles focus on how to best offer patient-centered care in *all* aspects of assessment, treatment, and ongoing care management, with appropriate and timely interprofessional communication, both for those in treatment and for survivors/thrivers.

What is a visit to a naturopathic doctor like? We conduct a full review of your health history as well as your current health status to gain a broad understanding of how your body's systems are functioning. We are also interested in any specific health concerns or worries you have, medications currently prescribed, and if you experience any side effects from those. We want to know which supplements and botanical medicines, if any, you currently take. We learn about your height and weight, your exercise history, as well as your diet, alcohol intake, smoking, recreational drug use, and other factors that influence your health. We want to understand what the main stressors are in your life and what strategies or tools you have for stress management.

We explore what your interest and capacity for lifestyle change is and what kind of resources you can allocate to your health. It's important that we understand such details: your ability for self-care, what sort of support you have, if any, and your willingness to re-prioritize certain aspects of your day-to-day life. A naturopathic doctor could create a detailed plan of recommendations, but if you cannot afford it, will not remember to do certain parts, or feel overwhelmed by the entire prospect, we'd need to reevaluate and modify a plan to your current capacity and ability. The health plans NDs create with and for you follow the strong philosophical base emphasized in naturopathic doctor training, as above.

The potential for and impact of collaborative work and research opportunities offer the best possible outcomes for patients. And of course, naturopathic doctors work with all kinds of patients, not just those who have had cancer. Over the last several decades there has been growing interest and training of other providers who are interested in learning natural and integrative medical approaches. The dominant medical paradigm is an enormous ship and is slowly turning toward preventive and natural medicine approaches. This is good for both individual and public health. Whatever your health concerns are, think about adding a naturopathic doctor or other provider trained in these approaches to your health-care team.

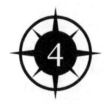

Macroenvironment, Microenvironment, and the Microbiome

MORE AND MORE research points to the *microenvironment* in and around tumor sites and how that environment impacts growth or spread of cancer. Think of it as its own ecosystem where all parts are interrelated and depend on one another to determine whether cancer will grow, go quiescent, or disappear. This microenvironment is extremely complex: the area contains a vast variety of immune-modulating cells, blood products, lymphatic tissue, communication channels, and all the surrounding material. Moreover, various features and factors of the microenvironment may be different in different areas of a cancerous site, yet all work together in a coordinated fashion.[16]

Think of a tree in the forest as the tumor. Everything around the tree—the soil, other plants, air and water nearby, access to sunlight (in other words, the *macroenvironment*)—influence how that tree grows and flourishes, or does not grow and dies. It's from the macroenvironment nourishing the microenvironment that a tumor will find all the necessary nutrients and substances it requires to create space for itself to multiply and grow. The more we learn about the tumor microenvironment, the more we grasp how it plays a role in the risk of developing cancer in the first place and the natural history of the illness. This understanding, in turn, can inform both preventive and treatment measures.[17]

Many of conventional oncology's effective treatments can increase the risk of developing other types of cancer. I remember signing consent forms during my cancer treatment that spelled out in black and white these potential side effects. At that time, I correctly understood the risk–benefit of chemotherapy, radiation, and targeted immunotherapy; while putting me at a small risk for other cancers in the future, they were essential and effective parts of my care. Knowing about the potential side effect of future cancer, along with the potential for metastasis of a current cancer, put my focus on what else I could do to *proactively* create an internal environment *least hospitable* to the development of new or returning cancer. The overall recommendations in this book are aimed right at this point.

Discussion and research on how to best manipulate the microenvironment to make it less hospitable to the development and spread of cancer is burgeoning.[18] Certain kinds of cancers have similar types of microenvironments, making it easier to specifically target treatments. The best approaches to date take into account how to aim at the blood supply nourishing cancer cells, or how to manipulate the overall immune system in the area, and/or how to employ tactics that work directly against cancer cells.

In addition, and especially pertinent for cancer survivors/thrivers, research points to the concept that a person's overarching macroenvironment influences the microenvironment related to the development, growth, and spread of cancer.[19] Variables that negatively influence the broader macroenvironment include a poor microbiome (see below), dysfunction in the neurotransmitter system from unrelenting stress, and the immunological impact from infections or traumatic events. Lifestyle choices and the greater external environment all play a role. Smoking, excessive alcohol intake, poor diet, being sedentary—all these and more create a less than optimal macroenvironment, which impacts your whole body as well as the microenvironment of any cancer cells. And, more to the point, for many of these physiologic functions, we have lifestyle or natural medicine modifiers to learn about, explore, and integrate into our lives for positive impact.

Below, I articulate general concepts, but there are also a number of natural medicine substances proven[20] to specifically influence the tumor microenvironment, to make it less hospitable to cancer cells trying to establish a tumor or spread. These include curcumin (*Curcuma longa*), the scientific name for the culinary herb turmeric; docosahexaenoic acid (DHA), an omega-3 fatty acid found in cold-water fish; epigallocatechin gallate (EGCG), found in green tea; resveratrol, found in the skin of red grapes, berries, and a number of other dark-skinned fruits; sulforaphane,[21] which has powerful antioxidant characteristics and is derived from leafy green vegetables, especially those in the *Cruciferae* family, like broccoli and kale; and vitamin D,[22] known for its many roles in overall immune function and in general healthy physiology. Each of these is described in more detail in chapter 7.

What are additional and broader ways to impact both the overarching macroenvironment and a tumor microenvironment? What do we know about normal physiologic activity that we can apply for best outcomes? Which dietary, lifestyle, and natural medicine tools have the most impact on making the least hospitable cancer environment? The answers to these questions make up the bulk of this book and are further delineated chapter by chapter. Suffice it to say that many natural medicine tools, both general and specific, work to create an optimal macroenvironment and microenvironment. Creating a robust and diverse microbiome is high on the list of goals to consider.

All this is to support a strong and balanced immune system.

The immune system is a marvelous, complex, agile, elegant, and essential part of the human body. Able to fight off infection, mount brave attacks on foreign entities, and recall previous biological insults in order to prevent them from coming back, the immune system performs amazing feats on a regular basis. It is also in charge of getting rid of unwanted cells, cells that may turn or become cancerous cells.

With the clarity of a sharpshooter, the immune system distinguishes between pathogens and unwelcome cells and a community of healthy cells. And sometimes it does not work as well as we want. When the immune system mounts a reaction to external exposures such as dust, dander, or particular foods, we have an allergy. If we take that continuum a little further, the immune system can go way overboard and begin to attack our own tissues and organs, wreaking havoc, which leads to autoimmune disease. And sometimes the immune system falls short in recognizing cancer cells and helping to stop their growth or spread. A well-functioning, alert, accurate, and effective immune system is always the goal. Likewise, immune therapies, increasingly studied and used in patient care, are receiving well-deserved attention and success.

The Microbiome

One of the most important aspects of appreciating your micro- and macroenvironments and supporting accurate immune function has to do with your microbiome. When I have the chance to listen to a full orchestra, I appreciate the fact that there are so many musicians playing different instruments, bringing out particular notes at the right tempo, with precise rhythm and intensity, each doing their part to create a full, rich, and multilayered sound. I think about the human microbiome similarly. On an even grander scale, the microbiome is made up of trillions of bacteria, viruses, and fungi along with genetic materials, working together in a multilayered way to promote health and well-being.

We have approximately ten times as many of these cells compared to human cells making up our bodies! We are indeed made of multitudes. While your microbiome is primarily in your gut, it exists throughout the body, too. A well-functioning microbiome supports effective digestion, sustains a responsive immune system, informs the maintenance of hormonal balance, impacts fertility for both men and women, and supports clear thinking and an even-tempered mood. The more it is studied,[23] the more we understand that a well-orchestrated microbiome plays a substantial role in the prevention of both acute and chronic illness, including cancer, and in fostering sound physical, cognitive, and emotional health.

A thriving microbiome is essential for digestion, absorption, and elimination. We also know[24] that a microbiome that is not working in concert with circadian rhythms has a negative impact on fat metabolism and weight gain. The gut microbiome affects how you absorb and metabolize nutrients and how you use your calories.

Addressing the microbiome has a positive impact on immune function, as there is a clear connection between the intestinal microbiome and the nervous system, which in turn is in constant communication with both the immune and hormonal systems. Studies[25] show the clear relationship between a robust and diverse microbiome and improved immune function. We also know that for some cancer therapies, including certain immunotherapies,[26] having a well-functioning microbiome has a clearly positive impact on health outcomes.

Dysbiosis is the term to describe a microbiome that is disturbed, which creates a more *pro-inflammatory* environment; among other negative impacts on health, this promotes the development, growth, or spread of cancer. Dysbiosis[27] is also associated with inflammatory bowel disease, metabolic disorder, obesity, depression, and other complaints.

What works against a healthy microbiome? This is where the macroenvironment comes in! Evidence[28] highlights how the impact of processed food, overprescription of antibiotics and other pharmaceuticals, and industrial farming, alongside other elements of modern times, have a grave impact on the extent and diversity of the human microbiome.

More broadly, the standard American diet (SAD) interferes with a balanced microbiome. SAD is defined by highly processed foods, refined carbohydrates and added sugars, hydrogenated fats, high-fat dairy products, and overeating red meat. Though many people know this would not make up a healthy diet, change can be difficult to embrace and sustain due to developed tastes, cultural factors, finances, and access to healthy foods.

Excessive alcohol consumption influences many aspects of physiology, including causing negative repercussions on the microbiome. Infectious disease can impact the function of the microbiome in its own ways. So, while the infectious disease might be helped by an antibiotic, the microbiome will also be further disturbed by antibiotics. See chapter 6 for more on eating right for an optimal microbiome.

Increasingly, the role of stress and the stress response and their impact on the microbiome are being examined.[29] Not surprisingly, intense or unrelenting stress has a negative impact on the health and balance of the microbiome. See chapter 11 on the head game for ideas and inspiration to help with stress reduction and stress management. Exercise should not be underestimated for its role in impacting both the macro- and microenvironment. Whatever else you do, remember that exercise should be at the top of your list of self-help approaches to create the least hospitable environment for cancer to flourish.

Here are some other ideas to consider:

Choose an anti-inflammatory diet. See chapter 6 for more information. When available and affordable, choose organic food. Sidestep foods you are allergic or sensitive to. If you drink alcohol, do so only in moderation.

Where you grew up and where you live now have an effect on your microbiome. Being in contact with the outdoors, with nature, and with dirt helps diversify your microbiome. Even just spending time in green spaces and outside can positively impact the microbiome.[30] Having an overemphasis on cleanliness may in fact *not* be working in our favor.

Toxic exposures in the environment cause many issues, including adding to the degradation of the microbiome, so work to decrease toxins as much as possible in your food and water, in your home, and in your personal care products. See chapter 14 for more ideas on how to minimize toxic exposures and better metabolize the exposures you have.

Taking a *probiotic* may well be worthwhile. One of the most common products in the food and supplements area, probiotics are defined as "live microorganisms which when administered in adequate amounts confer a health benefit on the host."[31] Generally recognized as safe, some studies reveal that probiotic content, consistency, and safety is not guaranteed. There is some evidence[32] of potential harm from probiotics, especially for those who are immune compromised from chronic ailments, AIDS, or chemotherapy. Be sure to work with your provider to determine if probiotics are indicated for you.

Many foods contain probiotic organisms, like fermented dairy in yogurt and kefir, soy products like miso and tempeh, some honey, fermented drinks like kombucha, fermented vegetables like sauerkraut, and the vast variety of the Korean condiment known as kimchi. You do not need to eat enormous quantities of these items; rather, include a small portion each day in your diet.

Prebiotics are the nondigestible fiber found in foods that help promote the growth of your microbiome. They provide nourishment for and are broken down by the microbiome in the digestive process. Prebiotics are a key area to consider when trying to improve your microbiome, and research[33] on prebiotics is rapidly growing. The products of that breakdown process include short-chain fatty acids, which are important for providing energy to our colon cells. They have broad impact across human physiology related to immune function, prevention of cancer,[34] and more.

Prebiotics are just as important as probiotics, though most people are able to ingest foods that provide adequate prebiotics. Eating a diet high in fiber will go a long way to providing the prebiotics your body needs. Foods with the best kind of prebiotic fiber include vegetables, fruit, whole grains, and legumes.

Our health, including our microbiome, is a product of our genetic inheritance, our lifestyle choices, and our environmental exposures. Some of us are more susceptible to falling ill, whether with an acute ailment, allergies, a chronic disease, or cancer. It is nearly impossible to escape our genes, though that may be less the case in the not-too-distant future!

Creating the healthiest possible internal environment can optimize our genetic predispositions. As the microbiome is developed, maintained, and influenced over the course of a lifetime, it works in an orchestrated and broad way. Knowing the microbiome exists, avoiding habits and exposures that impair its function, and tending to its health by improving its diversity and robustness are all worth your time. Your efforts may well have a far-reaching impact on your overall health and vitality. Approaches delineated in this book, from diet, exercise, and stress management to particular natural medicine tools, all start to make sense when appreciated within the context of both the macro- and microcellular environments.

Patient Story

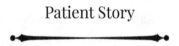

Some years ago, I had the opportunity to work with twelve-year-old Chad, who had undergone treatment for acute lymphoblastic leukemia. Like most children who go through that treatment protocol, he took prophylactic antibiotics. This helps to reduce the risk of serious bacterial infections, especially in the first key months of treatment.

I saw Chad about a year after his last round of chemotherapy. He handled his treatment well enough and had an excellent prognosis but was left with chronic diarrhea. Chad was a bright and outgoing child with a spark in his eye and an easy laugh. He told me the worst thing about the diarrhea was that it was unpredictable and the urge to go to the bathroom could come on quickly.

We worked first to address his diarrhea and also, as described above, to help create a healthier microbiome. I prescribed a high-strength, multi-organism probiotic. We explored the list of all the foods and drinks that are fermented/cultured and came up with some he really liked, including yogurt, kefir, and miso soup. I also used a number of botanical medicines to help soothe his irritated colon, including slippery elm (*Ulmus fulva*) and aloe vera juice. In addition, I recommended the amino acid glutamine, which helps create healthy mucous membrane lining of the bowel.

Within a week, Chad's diarrhea had improved, with both fewer bowel movements a day and more formed stool. By the end of two weeks, he was having one to two bowel movements a day and had lost any sense of urgency. Over the next few months, we discontinued the glutamine and reduced the probiotic to twice a week. I encouraged him to continue to include fermented foods in his diet.

Some ten years later, I continue to see Chad from time to time for other complaints, like acne, but he remains cancer-free with a healthy digestive system.

Exercise, Your New Best Friend

THE ROLE OF exercise and cancer survivorship has been thought about and studied, and the verdict is in. For most any person post-cancer, exercise is the number one modifiable action you can take to help improve both quality and length of life. I don't say this lightly, and I am not exaggerating: being sedentary is a changeable risk factor for your overall health. Let me explain why I believe that if you only change one behavior, you should begin to exercise, and if you already exercise, you should think about bumping it up a notch or two.

Research[35] shows that regular activity appears to *reduce the risk of all causes of death*, along with recurrence of cancer, while also preventing a number of other common illnesses such as obesity, cardiovascular disease, and diabetes. Long-term studies[36] show that consistent exercise improves quality of life. Exercise helps raise your threshold for feeling stress and helps dissipate stress you have. It also helps with perfusion (getting the blood moving), which amplifies the impact of many other conventional and natural medicine efforts you make.

There is growing evidence[37] that regular exercise helps address the often long-lasting fatigue many cancer survivors complain about. Exercise also builds back muscle mass,[38] helps maintains bone mass,[39] reduces cardiac toxicity,[40] and reduces oxidative stress, which, among many other attributes, helps you think more clearly. Exercise has also been shown to improve *the actual benefit* of many conventional cancer treatments. Exercise slows down cancer cell multiplication and helps promote *apoptosis*, or natural programmed cell death—one way our body gets rid of unwanted cells, including cancer cells.

Science[41] points to specific ways exercise helps to stop cancer cell growth, including improving the internal microenvironment around cancer cells; increasing overall blood flow throughout your body; encouraging the development of healthy blood vessels; reducing fasting levels of circulating blood sugar; stimulating innate immunity; reducing the stress hormones associated with cancer progression; and helping to address excess weight, a known risk factor for some cancers. While exercise is good for all patients in treatment and for all cancer survivors, evidence is most profound—likely because these cancers have been studied more—for improving both prognosis and survival for those with a history of prostate, colorectal, or breast cancer.

Cancer cells have been shown to be less aggressive when a person regularly engages in moderate exercise.[42] Exercise helps by correcting aberrant angiogenesis (the development of new blood vessels, including blood vessels to nourish cancer cells,) and stimulating immune function to attack circulating tumor cells, among other physiologic processes. In addition, hypoxia, which is an insufficient oxygen supply at the tissue level, *encourages* a cancer microenvironment and makes it easier for cancer cells to set up shop. Exercise is a key way to reverse the hypoxic microenvironment.

Endorphins, or happy hormones released with exercise, help with mood while also having a clear impact on your nervous system, which in turn impacts your immune system. We want to support immune capacity as much as possible, especially in its star anticancer role.

Some symptoms or situations may interfere with regular exercise, such as lymphedema, ostomy, and peripheral neuropathy and/or extreme fatigue, so you will need resources to address these situations. See chapter 17. If you've taken chemotherapy that is tough on your heart or lungs, you will want to be cleared for exercise before beginning a program, and modify as needed. And for those with low iron from treatment, you will have less energy and less endurance to start, but these are challenges that gradually improve over time for many people. If treatment caused weakness, if you've lost muscle mass, if your balance is off, start slowly and build your way up over time. Self-compassion and patience come in very handy.

It's good to think about exercise in three categories—aerobic, weight or resistance training, and flexibility exercises—and to consider how striving every week for some of each is important. I recommend that my patients get their exercise in the morning. For many people, if exercise is left to the end of the day, it may not happen. That said, the most important aspect is to create a routine that works with your schedule and stay with it. I know; easier said than done. But the scientific evidence to support the essential role of exercise for cancer survivors is exceedingly clear, so hopefully that will help with motivation!

Aerobic exercise, which you may hear called cardio, means literally "with oxygen." When you're doing this kind of exercise, you raise your breathing and heart rate, which is excellent for your heart, lungs, and circulatory system. It helps many other physical systems in a number of ways. You become better perfused, meaning your blood is moving around your body better. You remove accumulated metabolites or toxins more efficiently. And all the while, you bring nourishment to your cells, tissues, and organ systems.

Kinds of aerobic exercise include brisk walking, jogging,

running, elliptical machines, kayaking or canoeing, rowing machines, hiking, dancing, swimming, cycling, jumping rope, and aerobic circuits (where you rotate among squats, lunges, push-ups, dips, etc.). Some people love classes such as kickboxing, Zumba, or other sorts of dance. Really, anything that gets your heart pumping is what you're after. I find that music really helps me get moving. I love to rollerblade, and music is the perfect companion on the local rail trails near my home.

Weight training helps with maintaining or building muscle mass, sustaining bone density, and improving insulin sensitivity and glucose tolerance. It's important to ask for guidance and direction if you are new to weight training. You want to be lifting the right amount of weight the right number of times (reps). I love inviting patients, especially middle-aged and older women, into the world of resistance training. It's very satisfying, and you can see progress pretty quickly. My only caveat is that you should first learn correct posture, form, and appropriate-for-you weight amounts and repetition numbers, in order to prevent injury. It's a good idea to engage, if possible, a private trainer or teacher at a gym, or a friend who knows this area, and let them know you are just getting back into exercise after an illness; be sure your instructor is sensitive to and mindful of your potentially unique needs.

There are traditional weight-training tools such as dumbbells and weight machines. Elastic resistance training with tubes or Therabands has been shown[43] to offer the same benefits as other weight-training tools and devices. Some benefits of elastic resistance training include low cost, easy transportability, and the ability to use anywhere.

For those of you more experienced with resistance training, recall that it's good to mix up your workouts, to add weight or reps over time to keep the activity fresh and to give your muscles something new to work on.

Stretching exercises enable your joints and muscles to attain better range of motion and flexibility, and are also known to improve balance. With these attributes, stretching exercises can help to prevent falls and other injuries, reduce stiffness and pain, and help your posture and overall strength. Some people recall stretching exercises from their youth. Other approaches might come in the form of yoga or Tai Chi, Qigong, or an exercise-ball routine. Yoga in particular has been studied[44] as an adjuvant therapy for cancer care, and it has been found that patients "improved the physical and psychological symptoms, quality of life, and markers of immunity." I also think about stretching metaphorically; when you are flexible and more agile physically, you may also be more flexible and agile with your thinking, and more emotionally resilient.

For many of us, once an exercise routine is established, we actually look forward to it. And soon after you begin, you feel the positive impacts. An added benefit of regular exercise is the improved mental health it conveys. Exercise reduces anxiety and depression, builds confidence and focus, and supports digestion and sleep—which is all to say it is one key habit for physical, cognitive, and emotional health.

What if you are in that group of people that *hates* exercise? I have people like this in my practice who would rather do anything, and I mean *anything*, than exercise. I'd like to invite you to try something new. An activity entirely different so you have no associated bad memories. A dance class. Online yoga. Fencing. Circus arts. Or if you are in the position to, consider adopting a dog. Walking your dog twenty minutes once or twice a day counts!

If all else fails, use technology to your advantage. Use your cell phone's built-in pedometer or download an affordable pedometer app. Do some consciousness raising by checking your pedometer. If you walk 600 to 700 steps a day, set small achievable goals for yourself. Be sure you have well-fitted shoes with good arch support. Aim for 2,000 steps a day and see how you feel when you achieve that. Most people can, with some attention and dedication, work up to 6,000 to 7,000 steps a day, a good goal in any event.

We know that setting small goals, having someone to be accountable to, and receiving encouragement along the way can help establish an exercise habit. With some focus and commitment, most people can increase their exercise output. And as long as you're moving in the right direction, emphasis on the word *moving*, I am in favor of that.

For those who have a clear muscle and body memory of enjoyable times exercising, bicycling, working out, hiking in nature and so on, it will not be as hard to get back into the swing of things. You may feel disappointed in what you can accomplish compared to a previous stage, but focus on the positive, and have faith in your body's ability to get better and stronger over time. Some abilities might be compromised, but adjusting output, using assistive devices, and modifying postures in yoga, for instance, are all possible.

Taking a small group class with a patient and encouraging instructor might be for you. And working with an athletic trainer can be useful not just for weight training; many gyms have staff who will help you through an overarching routine that includes aerobics, stretching, and weight bearing. Some of us do better with one-on-one attention like that. In contrast, some of us use our exercise time to be on our own, to focus on our goals, to space out, to listen to a podcast. Whatever it takes!

Some patients on hormone treatment need to take special care of their bones and should prioritize weight-bearing exercise like walking, running, racquet sports, and weight training. Remember that swimming, though terrific for a full-body workout, relaxation, coordination, and cardiovascular health, is—alas—*not* weight bearing. If you love it but need to focus more on the weight-bearing piece, enjoy swimming one or two times a week and mix in other kinds of exercise. Bicycling is also not especially weight bearing (sorry). In fact, long-distance cyclists and swimmers are both known to have lower bone density than others, though they suffer fewer fractures, likely due to better coordination.

Patients ask me if it's okay to do the same exercise over and over. Is it important to get all three kinds of exercise? I emphasize that any exercise is important. If you go for a walk every day and it's the only thing you do for exercise, but you are consistent, enjoy it! If you are able to dip a toe into the other areas, I would be supportive, but really, *any* movement is good!

On a personal note, as a beneficiary of the first wave of Title IX, the 1972 federal civil rights law that expanded opportunities for women and girls in school athletics, I played three sports in high school. I gained skills and understanding about so much in life: the importance of teamwork, the commitment to discipline, learning to trust and lean on others, and knowing how to push past fear, difficult moments, and disappointment. I also learned how to be a gracious winner. I was an outside striker for the South Shore High School volleyball team in Brooklyn, which I enjoyed entirely. I miss SMASHING something . . . anything . . . to smithereens like that! I certainly learned about being in the moment and finding ways to get my head in the "zone" (more on that in chapter 11 on the head game), though I'm fairly certain that in 1976, we didn't call it that.

All these attributes of playing a team sport were a kind of preconditioning for my going through cancer treatment. Those same qualities, learned on a volleyball court decades ago, served me well during a more challenging time.

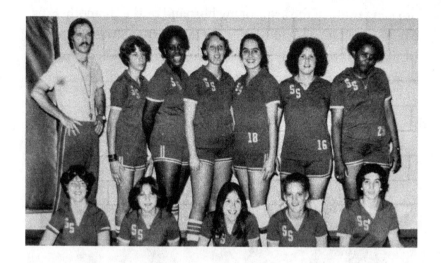

*Here I am, circa 1977, sporting #18 with my beloved
high school volleyball team.*

And in what could only be filed under the what-else-can-I-do-to-prevent-recurrence category, I completed my first triathlon six months after my last of eighteen rounds of chemotherapy. With my grown kids, husband, and extended family on board, we made it a family event, and, boy, did I feel triumphant crossing that finish line! Competing in that and many triathlons since then is testament to conventional and naturopathic medicine and my own stubborn belief that I'd come back better than ever. It continues to be helpful to have the goal of competing in those races to drive my already healthy discipline around exercise each year. Plus, it's fun to bring the family together on a mission.

I also began to learn the fine art of social ballroom dance[45] several years before my diagnosis. This exercise hit high marks for learning something new, for being aerobic and weight bearing, for improving flexibility, for social connection, as well as for the musical and sensual components. There were times during treatment when I was not sure what was doing me more good—an amazing waltz in the arms of my husband or the chemotherapy. My husband and I had been welcomed so generously into our local dance community, and those friendships and connections were an important part of my healing, which I will share more about in chapter 11.

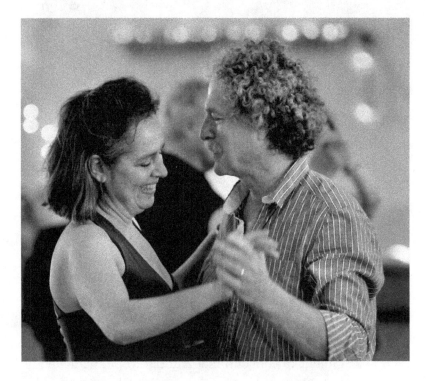

Dancing with my husband, 2018, photo by Kevin Gutting

The studies about exercise and cancer survivorship are many and varied, and they all pretty much come to the same conclusion. Most survivors can tolerate at least some exercise. You should take the exercise recommendation seriously; take time finding something you enjoy that is sustainable, where you won't get injured. Then, reorganize the taking-care-of-yourself to-do list so you bump exercise to the number one position.

Patient Stories

Larry, sixty-eight, a survivor of prostate cancer, was feeling pretty low after treatment was complete. He now had no prostate, was on hormone therapy, and came to me for help getting back on his feet. Once an avid racquetball player, he did not feel he'd be able to keep up with the intensity or endurance required of that sport. This was depressing to Larry, and I sensed his overall enthusiasm for life waning.

I knew Larry was a competitor and that he prided himself on his athleticism. I introduced him to the game pickleball, which is played on a half tennis court and requires much less running. He initially balked, but by the time I saw him again two months later, he could tell me everything about the game, the group he was playing with, and how pickleball felt like something normal, fun, and vigorous that helped his spirits. He also got back into the gym, where he felt like he was starting at the beginning; but with dedication and discipline, Larry was lifting weights and working to maintain his weight, his muscle mass, and his bone density.

Laura, age sixty, was never much of an exercise person. She had just completed treatment for colon cancer and came to see me for help recovering from her year of treatment and to try and prevent recurrence. As we spoke about many elements of a possible plan, it became clear that Laura was happy to work on her diet, bring meditation back into her life, and take a small selection of indicated nutritional supplements. But when I broached the topic of exercise, Laura told me flat out that she was not interested. She didn't have time to exercise, she didn't like to exercise, she hated to sweat, and, well, couldn't I help her with recommendations besides exercise?

I took time to review with her the evidence and paramount importance of exercise and how it would amplify every other change and effort she made. I listed some of the other benefits of regular exercise (more energy, better sleep, healthier-looking skin, etc.). She finally agreed to "try," and so we started very slowly. She committed to taking 2,000 steps a day, and much of that she would do inside her home. To me, this was not ideal, as I prefer some exposure to sunshine for vitamin D activation and for a change of scenery. But I realized I would have to pick my battles. Over the course of the next year, Laura realized that she actually felt better when she walked and had increased to 4,000 steps a day. She continued to resist weight training or anything related to stretching, but this was much better than nothing. Small steps to better health.

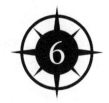

Diet and Nutrition, Intermittent Fasting, and Reaching Optimal Weight

SOME CANCER SURVIVORS have always eaten a healthy balanced diet, while some tend to be junk-food junkies. Most people I speak with are somewhere in the middle. Many tell me they know more or less what they *should* eat but do not always make good choices. It may be due to time constraints, resources, fatigue, less-than-stellar habits, or a psycho-emotional relationship to food and eating. What is the best diet for cancer survivors to regain health and stay healthy? What should you eat to reduce your risk of recurrence? This chapter shares broad-stroke recommendations in these departments on nutrition and eating.

Start by raising your consciousness about what you *do* eat. Keep a diet diary for a week, including a weekend. Then review it. If possible, enlist help from someone who understands nutrition. When you take an honest look back over a week's worth of vittles, you may see patterns like "I really do like my carbs!" Or "I guess I really don't take in enough veggies." Or "Geez, I didn't realize how much alcohol I drink." Sometimes we're pleasantly surprised, like "Hey, I get high points for my fruit intake." Being self-aware is the first step to shifting to a healthier diet. Once you decide to improve your diet, consider inviting a friend or family member to join you for healthier eating. Community and connection, trading ideas, swapping recipes, sharing a meal, and offering encouragement can go a long way toward helpful and enduring dietary changes.

Do you need a specialized diet? Patients often ask me about certain diets they have heard about, wondering if they're good ones to adopt. Researchers continue to examine which diets may be best for cancer patients and survivors, and the American Cancer Society (ACS) incorporates much of this research into their well-articulated dietary advice.[46] The basic ACS guidelines include the following: eat nutrient-dense foods that do not lead to weight gain; take in a variety of vegetables and legumes; eat several pieces of fruit per day; choose whole grains over refined grains; keep red meat and processed meat to a minimum; and sidestep both sugary drinks and excessive alcohol consumption. Most integrative cancer doctors embrace the ACS dietary advice and expand upon it, as I will do with recommendations below. But first let's consider a number of specialized diets, including the alkaline diet, ketogenic diet, vegetarian and vegan diets, and macrobiotic diet.

An alkaline diet is predicated on the idea that a less acidic internal environment will be less hospitable to cancer cells, their growth and spread. A strictly alkaline diet, including drinking alkaline water, has been studied extensively in people-based clinical trials and has consistently fallen short. That said, many of the components of an alkaline diet, such as eating more vegetables and limiting red meat, do show good effect. We need more studies on the alkaline diet.

The ketogenic diet, first developed for those with epilepsy, has also been examined for cancer.[47] The idea behind the ketogenic diet is to eat a very high-fat, low-carb diet where you burn fat instead of carbs for your main form of energy. This puts you in a state of ketosis, which has physiologic impacts, perhaps ones that are less hospitable to cancer. This diet has been tested both to see if it helps the efficacy of treatment and as another part of treatment for certain cancers, including an aggressive brain cancer, glioblastoma. It may help with decreasing overall inflammation. It may also help to keep weight from creeping up, which is a risk factor for some cancers. It may be pertinent for the prevention of metastasis for other cancers.

There is conflicting research on the ketogenic diet, however. For instance, it relies heavily on meat, which is associated with an increase in cancer incidence. The keto diet also requires continual measurement of fats, carbs, and protein, which can be challenging to sustain. And while it shows promise for certain people with particular cancers, it is contraindicated for those with a history of eating disorders, digestive disturbance, kidney stones, or extreme weight loss. If you are interested in exploring the ketogenic diet, please only do so under careful guidance from a qualified provider.

Vegetarian and vegan diets both show protective effects on general health. This is especially true if there are limits on refined carbohydrates, refined sugars, fried food, and alcohol. For some people who have had a hard time with wound healing or who have muscle-mass loss, eating an animal-free diet may contribute to those challenges. We need more studies on both specific and general impact of vegetarian and vegan diets for cancer survivors.

The macrobiotic diet is based on a philosophical approach that takes into consideration your gender, activity level, climate, and season of the year. It is plant-based and almost opposite to a ketogenic diet, relying mostly on complex carbohydrates, low fat, and plant-based foods. Elements of the diet fall under my general recommendations of eating organic foods and taking in a lot of vegetables as well as fish. Although it has been a popularized as an anticancer approach, no clinical trials or evidence show the macrobiotic way of eating will help to prevent or treat cancer.

It's important to remember that no one diet will work for everyone, and I encourage you to appreciate the concept of biochemical individuality. Naturopathic doctors have advanced training[48] in nutrition, and I aim to put it to good use when making personalized dietary recommendations to my cancer patients/survivors. Here are my general suggestions pertinent to most survivors:

✦ **EAT FOOD.** I know this sounds odd, but I have many patients who, in their drive to eat well, shift over to instant shakes and bars, often eaten standing at the kitchen counter or on the run. While some of these items are not terrible, I emphasize eating whole, recognizable food. Similarly, eat food that is less processed. Fresh is best; frozen is second best! If you cannot understand something on a label, you probably should leave it on the shelf.

✦ **REMOVE FOOD ALLERGENS FROM YOUR DIET.** Inflammation[49] in the body is associated with cancer progression, and eating foods to which you are sensitive or allergic can cause and contribute to inflammation. Some people have a sense that they do not react well to a certain food, as in "Every time I eat dairy, I have loose stools," or "I love eggs, but they don't love me!" I recommend you start by removing those foods. After that, consider food-allergy or food-sensitivity testing. The difference between a food allergy and sensitivity is how your body responds to the offending food. If you have a food allergy, the reaction comes from your immune system and is measured by levels of an immunoglobulin, a type of antibody in your blood, called IgE. Symptoms can be anywhere on your body, from hives and other skin reactions to swelling and itching. If instead you have a food sensitivity or a food intolerance, reactions are usually limited to the digestive system in the form of gas, bloating, and indigestion. Food sensitivities are measured by levels of IgG—a different kind of immunoglobulin—in your blood.

While you may do better off of some foods, it's also true that as you regain health and work on developing a robust and diverse microbiome, you may find that some foods that previously caused problems are better tolerated. For some of my patients, portion size comes into play. In other words, if they are sensitive to, say, dairy, they may be able to have a small portion once or twice a week without concern.

✦ **BUMP UP THE VEGETABLES COUNT.** There is good and mounting evidence[50] that it's not just the amount but rather the *variety* of vegetables eaten that has a protective effect. Here are two of the easiest ways to increase your vegetable intake: include one or two vegetables with breakfast, and eat one salad a day. My go-to breakfast is steamed or sautéed onion, garlic, and kale scrambled with eggs or tofu. Sometimes I have steamed vegetables and rice with a poached egg, or oatmeal with a side of steamed carrots. I have let go of the concept of what constitutes a breakfast food. Liberating! The other trick I use is to keep frozen organic vegetables in my freezer. While I often have time to peel, cut, chop, cook, and clean, sometimes I do not. A quick steam stovetop is very easy and still counts. For my salad, I include five, six, or seven vegetables in the bowl, which I take to work or eat at home. I often purchase prewashed lettuce as I find I use it more if I don't have to wash it. As a grateful member of a local community-supported agriculture project, I enjoy greens from the farm in season. I love to grate beets, carrots, radishes, and red cabbage onto my salad. I add more typical fare, such as tomatoes and cucumber. I add some form of protein like a hardboiled egg, leftover grilled chicken or salmon, legumes or nuts, then a healthy drizzle of olive oil, a dash of either lemon juice or vinegar, a forkful of fermented vegetables— and there's my tasty, nutritious salad. By eating another one or two vegetables with dinner, I have reached a goal I set for myself of eight to ten vegetables a day. I do not reach that goal every day, but having a goal directs my hand when I open the fridge or order at a restaurant. Often when I eat out, regardless of what I am ordering, I will ask for the vegetable of the day as a side order, steamed, no salt.

✦ **STOP OR SERIOUSLY REDUCE ALCOHOL INTAKE.** Research[51] shows that the more you drink, the more at risk you are for developing certain kinds of cancer. Many of my patients ask me what's a safe amount of alcohol to ingest on a regular basis. The answer is (sadly) zero! That said, a glass of wine with dinner or a cold beer on a hot summer day, once in a while, will not cause cancer, so feel free to enjoy it, as long as you are not an alcoholic.

✦ **TAKE FAST FOODS OUT OF YOUR DIET.** They are typically loaded with salt, hydrogenated fats, and simple carbohydrates. If you are in a pinch, see if you can order whatever salad is available, and no matter how tempting it is, don't get the fries!

✦ **EAT CULTURED FOODS EACH DAY.** There is emerging evidence[52] that a robust and diverse microbiome is relevant for overall physical, emotional, and cognitive health. Eating naturally fermented sauerkraut, pickles, kimchi, miso, yogurt, kefir, and the many cultured foods that various places around the world offer, helps to diversify your gut flora. In turn, this helps support optimal immune function. About 80 percent of your immune system arises from your gut, and you're dependent on your immune system to do all its broad-reaching jobs. For more information on the role of the microbiome and cancer, see chapter 4. To further elucidate the role of the microbiome in mental and cognitive health, see chapter 11 on the head game.

✦ **REDUCE SUGARS AND CARBOHYDRATE INTAKE.** Studies[53] show that overeating these foods and having a high glycemic load is associated with poorer outcomes. By reducing refined sugar, we make our bodies more sensitive to insulin, and this helps to reduce inflammation, one known trigger for cancer. In general, eat as if you were a type 2 diabetic: avoid high-glycemic foods, including white bread, most other white-flour-based foods, and white potatoes. Allow yourself one or two small pieces of dark chocolate each day, if you like it, as that does good[54] work in your body as a potent antioxidant!

✦ **EAT ALL THE BERRIES YOU LIKE.** Except for the cost, this should not be hard to do as they are tasty, with no known side effects and with good evidence[55] to support their anticancer impact. Ditto for dark grapes.[56] The same can be said of berry juices, which are jam-packed with antioxidants. They are high in sugar, however, so dilute juices with water or sparkling water, and limit yourself to a half to one cup a day.

✦ **EAT HEALTHY FIBER AND PREBIOTICS.** Eat whole grains, such as brown rice and quinoa, as well as legumes and fresh fruit to ensure a healthy intake of fiber and prebiotics, both essential for a well-tended digestive tract able to absorb and integrate nutrients, support regular elimination, and maintain a healthy microbiome.

✦ **EAT NUTS.** Walnuts and other nuts are an excellent source of healthy fats, fiber, and protein and offer other anticancer benefits.[57] A nut portion should be about the number of nuts that fit in the palm of your hand. In other words, don't sit down with a whole bag of nuts; that is too many calories for most people.

✦ **EAT SOY FOODS.** Soybeans[58] and related foods, such as tofu, tempeh, and soy milk, should also be included in the diet. Misinformation has spread about soy putting people more at risk of breast cancer. There is no evidence of that. In fact, post-treatment, eating soy is associated with better health outcomes.

✦ **INCLUDE HEALTHY OILS.** Oils to include on a regular basis are olive oil,[59] coconut oil, and avocado oil, all boasting anticancer influence. They also add flavor and help with a sense of satiety. Consider trying and including ghee in your diet. Ghee is clarified butter, and through the Ayurvedic tradition it has been used for millennia to excellent effect on many systems of the body. I like to spread ghee on gluten-free toast but also use it in cooking, and it is especially delicious in soups and stews.

✦ **DRINK POMEGRANATE JUICE.** Drinking three to four ounces per day provides anticancer effects.[60] Remember that fruit juices have a lot of sugar, which can be inflaming, so dilute with water or sparkling water or green tea[61] if you like. While pomegranates and pomegranate juice offer many health benefits, it may, like grapefruit juice, interfere with some medications, so please consult your provider before including in your diet.

✦ **DRINK GREEN TEA.** Drink a cup of green tea each day if you like it. Find the decaf green tea if you have insomnia, hypertension, bladder issues, or anxiety. You can mix with other teas for flavor, as you prefer.

✦ **EAT AND BAKE WITH FLAXSEEDS.** There is plenty of research[62] to support eating one to two tablespoons of ground flaxseed a day for its anticancer role. Grind it yourself in a coffee or nut grinder or buy it already ground and keep it in the freezer so it won't go rancid. Put in yogurt or oatmeal or add it to a smoothie. You can also use it in many baking recipes.

✦ **COOK AND SEASON WITH GINGER ROOT,[63] TURMERIC ROOT,[64] GARLIC AND ONIONS,[65] CINNAMON,[66] AND USE MUSHROOMS WHEN YOU CAN.** These all have an anticancer impact. Examination[67] of healing components of many culinary mushrooms point to impressive results.

✦ **WHAT ABOUT COFFEE?** If you like it, enjoy it! Studies report,[68] at least for breast cancer survivors, that coffee intake reduces all-cause mortality. And two to three cups are better than one, reducing mortality by a whopping 26 percent. Caffeinated had a slightly better impact than decaf, but decaf also offered protection. It turns out that coffee is an excellent antioxidant and, as might be predicted, the most common source of antioxidants in the American diet. Remember to limit the refined sugars and sweetened milks used in your coffee. Also, if you have bladder issues, anxiety, insomnia, palpitations, or GERD, coffee may well be contraindicated. Consider drinking a tall glass of water before your coffee, as coffee can be dehydrating. Also consider drinking your coffee with food so it will be less hard on your stomach.

✦ **LIMIT RED MEAT.** Choose fish, poultry, or beans instead of beef, pork, and lamb, whenever you can. If you eat red meat, aim for smaller portions and lean cuts. Use organic, grass-fed meats if you can afford it. Eggs are fine!

✦ **ELIMINATE PROCESSED MEAT.** Avoid processed meats such as hot dogs, ham, beef jerky, and deli meats. The World Health Organization has tagged the entire group[69] as carcinogenic.

✦ **REDUCE SODIUM INTAKE.** This is especially important if you've had stomach cancer.[70] Aim for less than 2,400 mg per day, which is about one teaspoon of salt. Start reading labels on prepared food (crackers, bread, chips, etc.), and you'll see how quickly you can rack up milligrams of sodium. When eating out, always request no added salt.

Salt brings out other flavors and, well, is often a desired taste! But as you reduce your sodium intake, your taste buds will adjust over time. If you go with limited salt for some weeks or months, many typically seasoned dishes will taste *too* salty.

✦ **BE MINDFUL.** Remember to eat seated at a table as often as possible. Put away your phone or computer. Light a candle. Say a little something to yourself or dining partner to ground you a bit before welcoming nourishment. Yes, the foods are important, but the attitude, the environment, the pace, the presence of mind, and gratitude may be equally important ingredients, especially when trying to attain optimal health. If you slow down enough to notice your food, you also aid digestion as the digestive enzymes have more chance to do their essential jobs.

✦ **GO SLOW, AND GO EASY ON YOURSELF.** Some of my patients are good at food shopping and stocking most of the foods they need. They can look in the fridge and the cupboard and pull together healthy, satisfying meals from what they find. Others need more encouragement and support. I don't care where a patient starts with their diet. I am happy to work with them or send them to a trusted colleague to help generate logical shopping lists and weekly menu plans that take into account lifestyle, budget, cultural elements, and food preferences. I keep a running list of favorite and healthy recipes[71] in many categories on my author website.

Remember, it's a rare day that anyone can integrate all these suggestions, unless they make shopping, cooking, eating, and cleaning up a full-time pursuit. My intention here is to list a range of foods and to underscore the research that supports eating certain ways and specific foods. But be realistic, pace yourself, and make slow, gradual shifts, which tend to be more enduring.

I also spend time brainstorming with patients about eating out, which can be a fun, social, "normal" activity that they look forward to continuing or getting back to after cancer treatment. And many of my patients travel for work or pleasure or both. How can you make good choices when you eat out, and how can you stay healthy on the road while also exploring unfamiliar, local cuisine? These are all conversations I welcome. We have fun brainstorming pertinent ideas. I always say that your body reflects the habitual, not the occasional. So once in a while, enjoy whatever looks good and you have a hankering for, as long as the usual fare arcs toward healthier!

My take-home advice to patients who have completed treatment is to eat a healthy-for-you, anti-inflammatory diet, as described above, and continue to adjust and alter as time goes on. Add in the foods and drinks as above, guided by your tastes and how adventuresome you're feeling. It remains ever true—we are what we eat. Use food as your first medicine. Bon appetit!

Intermittent Fasting

You've read about *what* to eat to regain and maintain health after cancer treatment. Now let's highlight *when* to eat, or in fact when to abstain, which, as evidence mounts, is just as important.

Naturopathic doctors have long advocated for the role of fasting in disease reversal and health maintenance. There are many types of fasting, from water fasting to juice fasting, to alternate-day fasting, to periodic fasting, to intermittent fasting.

The health impacts of caloric restriction or having longer stretches of time without eating are numerous. Research[72] shows a broad and positive impact on health, including prevention of cardiovascular disease, inflammatory illnesses, obesity, *and* cancer.

When I was in chemotherapy treatment, I ate a restricted 800-calorie vegan diet the two days before, the day of, and the day after chemo. The idea was that healthy cells can go many days without ample nourishment, where cancer cells cannot. By restricting intake, I weakened any cancer cells that were around, hence making the chemo more effective. One positive effect of such caloric restriction, which many of my patients also report, is fewer symptoms from the chemotherapy: less nausea, fatigue, and overall discomfort. Like all medicine, this approach is not for everyone and must be tailored to the individual. Let me emphasize: *if you have a history of disordered eating or are already underweight, quite weak, or you have dangerously low blood counts, this would not be recommended during chemotherapy.*

For those who have completed treatment or who are living well enough with cancer, intermittent fasting may well have the capacity to tune up the immune system and support pathways that help fight cancer. Studies[73] show that an elongated overnight fast helps with both glucose regulation and with quality of sleep, both important for good health. When we fast, our cells also initiate an inherent repair process, including autophagy,[74] where older and less functional cells are removed.

Listed here are three fasting approaches my patients use *after* conventional care to optimize health and to help create an internal environment less hospitable to cancer. For that matter, I have many patients *at risk* for cancer, heart disease, and/or diabetes who have adopted intermittent fasting as another important element of preventive care.

Eat freely five days a week, but for two days a week (no need to be consecutive), take in only 800 calories. This works well for people who are disciplined and don't mind the restrictiveness and impact on social eating.

Or for three to four consecutive days, once a month, keep your dietary intake in the 800-calorie range. This can work well for those able to carve out this much time, lighten their workload or family responsibilities, and enjoy a more inward time of reflection and quiet.

Another option, which I have both recommended and practiced for years now, is intermittent fasting: eating all your food within an eight-to-ten-hour period of the day, say 9 a.m. to 6 p.m., or in my case more like 11 a.m. to 7 p.m. In essence, I fast for thirteen to fourteen hours within each twenty-four-hour period. Whenever I finish dinner or a nighttime snack, I look at the clock. I know I will have breakfast in fourteen hours. I prefer patients not go to bed hungry, because that can interfere with deep, restorative sleep.

The easiest way to take on the elongated overnight fast is to first become aware of your current habits. Keep track of when you last eat and when you first eat for a week without trying anything new. If you snack at 10 p.m. and have breakfast at 7 a.m., you have a nine-hour overnight fast. The sweet spot for best impact seems to be in that thirteen-to-fourteen-hour range, so it would be arduous to make such a jump from, say, eight to thirteen hours. Take time over the course of months by stopping your intake of food thirty to sixty minutes earlier in the evening or having breakfast thirty to sixty minutes later in the morning. If you go slowly, you will have success. Many of my patients report that by the end of one week on the new schedule, they have adjusted and do not find it too arduous. And then over the course of months, you can continue to lengthen your overnight fast.

If you mess up one day—say there's a later social gathering or an early-morning business breakfast—it does not matter. Just pick up the next day. Many people report that the earlier they stop eating, the less hungry they are in the morning. By the way, black coffee does not count, so you can start out with your "cuppa joe," just with no sugar or any kind of milk. I know this flies in the face of what we've heard about breakfast being the most important meal, and that may well be true, but no one said *when* you had to eat it!

Intermittent fasting enhances insulin sensitivity, which in turn reduces inflammation, which has anticancer impact. Research[75] is mounting to support this effort, and it adds zero cost with nary a side effect—except the many other health benefits. Many people lose weight without trying. The total number of calories you eat in the day may not be reduced, but you make better use of the calories you take in. Many of my patients report feeling better self-control and self-agency, which trickles over into other aspects of life, such as getting regular exercise and ensuring adequate sleep. When you make one good lifestyle choice, it often spawns others. I love to hear from patients about their positive spiral of health based on new or reinvigorated healthy lifestyle choices.

Reaching Optimal Weight

Studies[76] increasingly show that being overweight is associated with worse outcomes related to survivorship. And it remains ever true that it can be difficult for some people to attain and maintain a healthy weight. Many factors go into being overweight. Primary among them are your genes, which, at least at this point, are predetermined. Add to that the environment you grew up in, food choices, exercise habits, and the impact of environmental factors, only some of which we can control. After thirty-six years of practice as a licensed naturopathic doctor, I can tell you that some people just cannot lose weight. They may have come to it genetically, they may have yo-yo dieted for decades, but the truth remains: they weigh more than they want to, and the extra pounds impact many elements of health and well-being, both physical and psychological. And for cancer survivors this presents even more of a challenge because being overweight influences health outcomes.

We used to think it was a mathematical equation, where eating less plus exercising more equaled gradual and permanent weight loss. While what you eat and how much you move are certainly relevant, scientific understanding of fat metabolism, the physiology of satiety, and the broad effect of a wide range of environmental chemicals on our hormones continues to evolve. We are learning about the many other important, ubiquitous factors at play. Our understanding of metabolism and how it changes over the course of a lifetime is becoming clearer too. From age twenty to about sixty, our metabolism, in fact, does not change measurably; only after that time does it begin to slow down until the end of life.

Adult women need around 1,600 to 2,400 calories per day. Adult men need between 2,000 and 3,000 calories. It used to be thought this was because men have faster metabolisms than women, but rather it's due to the fact that men on average have more muscle and less fat than women, and muscle uses up more energy (or calories) than fat. Somewhere between 55 to 70 percent of calories we take in go to powering the myriad of essential and invisible chemical reactions in our bodies that occur without much thought or encouragement in order to keep us alive.

There are many obstacles to losing weight. They are as unique and individual as a person's temperament or physical symptoms might be. This is because of the ever-important concepts of *biochemical individuality and susceptibility,* where all manner of factors influence people differently. These include genetic inheritance, lifestyle choices, events experienced throughout life, environmental exposures, underlying constitutional state, and more.

Rates of obesity in the United States are soaring at 42 percent of the adult population, climbing over 40 percent for the first time in our history, according to the *State of Obesity: Better Policies for a Healthier America*[77] by Trust for America's Health. Since 2008, this indicates a 26 percent increase in national adult obesity. Childhood obesity rates are also skyrocketing; over 19 percent of youths between the ages of two and nineteen are considered overweight; many will struggle with weight issues for the rest of their lives. We have a dire trajectory if the numbers continue in this direction and at this pace. For those with other risk factors for developing cancer, this is an added concern.

Like many health disparities, the statistics around obesity are astounding. Those with more money and more education tend to be thinner. Those living in rural communities develop more obesity, and people of color, wherever they live, on average are more overweight. Like other complicated, health-related challenges, the solutions are multilayered and span many areas, including environmental advocacy, city planning, health-care delivery, early education, the role of stress, and the uneven distribution of access to healthy foods.

Being overweight causes its own problems for some people, like low self-esteem or difficulty with mobility, and also predisposes people to a raft of common and serious diagnoses, including type 2 diabetes, hypertension, infertility, stroke, and sadly, certain cancers.

For people trying to lose weight, here are my top recommendations:

Elongate your overnight fast, as described above. A 2021

study[78] showed that beginning a weight loss effort with several days of restricted calories helps to jump-start weight loss, lowers blood pressure, and reduces other inflammatory markers in the blood. One reason this happens is because your microbiome is altered, engendering an environment more favorable for weight loss. Added benefits of intermittent fasting for many people include more discipline, lower appetite, and increased feelings of satiety. Giving your digestive system a break also allows other areas of physiology, like immune function, time for more focused and effective work.

Eat an anti-inflammatory diet. Though most people know this intuitively, it remains important to lean away from foods that are high in calories but low in nutrients, like candy, soda, and packaged snack foods. We'd all do better to eat more vegetables, fruit, nuts and seeds, lean proteins, cultured and fermented foods, and healthy fats. This basic anti-inflammatory diet decreases inflammation in general, and helps with lowering weight.

Inflammation is often part of the issue in those who cannot lose weight. When people eat a diet that emphasizes refined grains and soda, meat and processed meat, they have many more circulating inflammatory chemicals called *cytokines* in the bloodstream. While cytokines serve many roles in the body, they also reflect an inflammatory state. Cytokines alter your body's insulin response. If you are more resistant to insulin, your pancreas makes more of it, and this stimulates the storage of fat. And those with insulin resistance have a tendency to put on more fat in the abdominal area. Such belly fat is linked to higher incidence of certain cancers, like esophageal, colon, and pancreatic cancer.

Inflammation throughout the body can also impact leptin, which is a little-mentioned hormone that helps with the sensation of satiety. Many of my patients tell me that they just don't feel full and so they keep eating until they do. For some, this has more of a psycho-emotional root cause, but for all, lowering overall inflammation throughout the body will improve the functioning of leptins, which in turn will help with a more appropriate sensation of satiety.

Inflammation also increases water retention, another aspect of weight gain for many people. Adopting or improving upon an anti-inflammatory diet, for all its many health benefits, including weight loss, makes good sense.

Nurture your microbiome. Studies[79] show that taking probiotics and prebiotics may positively influence hormonal production and secretion as well as neurotransmitters—which, among other roles, impact hunger, appetite, satiety, and weight. Building a beneficial microbiome plays a key role in attaining a good-for-you weight.

Keep moving. Remember that aerobic exercise remains an essential piece of reaching and staying at your optimal weight. Walking counts! Online dance or exercise classes can work. Taking the steps in your apartment building for exercise can do in a pinch. The key is to find a time each day to fit in at least a half hour of aerobic activity. And then through the rest of the day, be mindful of too much sitting around, in front of the computer or the television. Being active throughout the day, taking stretching breaks, doing a few jumping jacks, or turning on some music and dancing in the kitchen all help to lower the negative impacts of a sedentary lifestyle. Read more on exercise in chapter 5 for information and inspiration.

Do what you can to ensure adequate sleep. Insufficient length of and poor-quality sleep may cause the intake of extra calories and certainly adds to fatigue, which leads many to poorer food choices and less motivation for exercise. Review chapter 12 for recommendations on sleep support.

Look at your stress and anxiety levels. Many people's stress level is off the charts. As stress mounts, so do cortisol levels, which increase insulin levels, which cause an increase in cravings for fatty and sweet foods. Read chapter 11 on the head game for information and ideas about how to reduce stress and, more importantly, how to reduce your *stress response*, which often lasts well beyond the actual or common stressors in your life.

Engage others in your efforts. Consider working up a weight-loss strategy with a friend or family member that you can do together. Clearly, the person needs to be someone you relate to, enjoy participating in similar activities with, and who is encouraging and supportive. It is often easier to break down larger problems into smaller ones and strategize together, celebrating small wins and being there for each other when you fall short. We all need help and support sometimes, and it is no different for weight loss.

Consider using technology to your advantage. A number of apps combine dietary recommendations, exercise suggestions, and mindfulness efforts, along with tracking capacity and a hefty dose of encouragement. A number of my patients have found success using technology to support change-making.

Obesogens

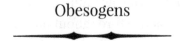

One factor not often described that can make it difficult for so many people to lose weight is the presence of obesogens in our diets and in our environment, both at home and out in the world. Obesogens are chemicals in our food, water, air, and household and personal products found in numerous forms, at startling rates, throughout our homes and outdoor spaces. As obesogens are increasingly studied,[80] we've gained a more comprehensive understanding of how their ubiquity is at least partly to blame for galloping rates of obesity across the world.

Obesogens are hormone disrupters, which means they can

alter the creation, secretion, capacity, and metabolism of the many hormones that go into overall normal human physiology. Obesogens were first studied for their impact on reproductive systems in the animal world, but as studies multiply, the far-reaching ways[81] obesogens influence health, in every system of the body, are becoming increasingly clear.

Obesogens impact metabolism and weight by changing the way fat cells develop and by increasing energy storage in fat tissue. They also disrupt the biochemical oversight of appetite and satiety and impact the variety and strength of the microbiome. Robust research[82] into how obesogens impact human health show they influence physiology by acting similarly to innate hormones, by binding to receptors in various parts of fat and other cells. This impacts the way a cell responds or the way a gene in the cell is expressed.

Many of the actions and alterations[83] obesogens cause are considered to be lifelong and, more alarmingly, passed down to subsequent generations. Women hoping to become pregnant or during pregnancy should take special care to reduce exposures as much as possible because of obesogens' potential impact on both fertility and the health of the baby. Obesogens may well change metabolic set points and lead to being overweight early in life, a risk factor for a lifelong struggle with weight.

Some exposures to obesogens are difficult to control and fall better in the realm of environmental action. But we *can* decrease exposure and would do well to do so, as time and resources allow. Of course, many of these items described are also associated with the incidence of cancer,[84] so reducing our overall toxin load in general, including obesogens, makes good sense. You can delve further into this topic in chapter 14 where I have listed the most common hormone disruptors and toxic chemicals, and how to try to avoid them in order to lower your overall toxic load.

Obesity is one of our largest national public-health crises, long in the making, without easy, enforceable strategies to counter. Using the precautionary principle, we should all be trying as best as we can to limit our and our family's exposures to obesogens in the home and in the environment. Consider becoming involved, as your time and bandwidth allow, with organizations that address environmental issues in your community and beyond. Active prevention is more effective than treatment for most all of our chronic diseases, including being overweight and developing cancer.

I would be remiss here to omit thoughts on the issues opposite to obesity. Some cancer patients and survivors struggle with keeping weight *on*. Cachexia, when the body goes overboard in breaking down skeletal muscle and fat stores in the adipose tissue, can be difficult to treat. Signs include low appetite, easy and early satiety, and signs and symptoms of malnutrition. This can be part of progressive illness and should be managed by a team approach that includes medications, nutrition, exercise, and counseling, as indicated. There are natural medicine approaches to consider, from appetite stimulation to nutritional supplementation, but this one requires more individualized and urgent attention, so please work with a qualified provider if this is your condition.

As being overweight is a modifiable though often challenging risk factor, whatever you can do to get to and stay at a healthier-for-you weight is worth the effort. Slow, gradual, and enduring changes are best and offer a long list of other health benefits. I have many patients in my practice who took their experience of a cancer diagnosis and treatment as a wake-up call to address many health issues, including being overweight, perhaps something they'd been ignoring or struggling with for years. I am always happily surprised and encouraged when I see patients take charge, make change, and enjoy the benefits they reap.

Patient Stories

When I first met Jennifer, she was eating a standard American diet—high in refined carbohydrates, simple sugars, fast foods, prepared foods, and sweets. She was the mother of two small kids and had just been through a bout of breast cancer. She came to me knowing she needed to tidy up her diet but overwhelmed by the prospect and not knowing where to start. We began with her keeping a one-week diet diary with what and how much food she ate and when she ate it.

I then asked Jennifer if some things in her diet were nonnegotiable. I often ask that question up front because I appreciate that food choices may carry enormous emotional content. She said right away that she could not eat fish. It disgusted her, and if I was going to ask her to eat fish, it just wouldn't work. I could live with that! I am much more interested in focusing on what people *should* eat instead of what they shouldn't eat. She committed to one salad a day to start. And she promised to cut back her diet cola habit by limiting it to only one a day from the typical three or four.

These were good starts, especially because we have learned that artificial sweeteners are very bad for health. Over the course of several visits, Jennifer and I carved out a diet she could live with. She tried some new items, including fermented foods and fruit-sweetened jams, and she was very pleased both with how she felt and by the fact that this was a healthier diet for a cancer survivor.

Another patient, Greg, came to see me soon after he completed treatment for leukemia. He had not felt very well during chemotherapy, so we decided it was too stressful a time to make many dietary changes. We focused our early visits on naturopathic approaches to insomnia, a new symptom for him (see chapter 12), and set our sights to work on his diet in the coming months. He felt he ate pretty well but wanted to know how else he could regain his strength while at the same time reducing his chance for recurrence.

A few months later, he was very keen to try the elongated overnight fast, as he was someone who often snacked until bedtime at 11 p.m. and had breakfast soon after waking at 7 a.m. I was confident that he could start stretching that fasting time and that he would adapt. He felt it was easier to push breakfast later, so he began by enjoying an early cup of coffee and eating breakfast an hour later. Within three months, Greg was at a consistent twelve-hour overnight fast, which he said made him feel more alert and more disciplined about getting his exercise. We have continued to work together on diet and other approaches to help him stay healthy and energetic.

Amanda came to me post-treatment for uterine cancer. She'd had a complete hysterectomy and radiation treatment to her abdomen. At five foot three, she weighed 160, which put her body mass index at a little over twenty-eight, which is considered overweight. She had struggled with weight her whole life. She carried her weight in her chest and belly, with thin arms and legs. She had not dieted much in her life; she mostly tried to lose weight by exercising and skipping desserts. She had time during her healing and recovery to put more effort into weight loss and was looking for recommendations. She felt an addiction to carbs was her downfall. She loved anything from the bakery—bread, donuts, bagels—as well as pasta. The more she ate it, the more she wanted it. She was prediabetic, according to her fasting blood sugar levels and her hemoglobin A1C levels, and she knew her diet was not helping.

She did have a good relationship with exercise and had some walking buddies she met with each week. Amanda also enjoyed in-person and online aerobic classes from her local gym.

I decided to run food-sensitivity tests for her as she was someone who put a lot of stock into knowing what was going on inside her body. She felt like if she had clear information, she might feel more motivated to make necessary changes.

As it turned out, Amanda was sensitive to gluten, soy, and citrus. In a paradoxical way, this was a relief for Amanda, and she immediately went to work removing gluten, which made up an enormous portion of her diet. There was gluten in most every meal and most of the snacks Amanda ate. I cautioned Amanda to not simply replace gluten products with gluten-free ones, as many of those are also quite high in carbs, or more specifically, refined carbohydrates. I encouraged her to try whole grains like brown rice, quinoa, and millet.

I also convinced Amanda about the essential role of fresh fruits and vegetables—that by increasing those, she'd also be increasing the fiber in her diet. Fiber would help support good elimination and feelings of satiety. We set the bar low because this would be the biggest change for her. She committed to including two pieces of fruit and three vegetables into her daily intake. She did not always hit this mark, but she had the goals in mind.

Amanda immediately starting losing weight, which inspired other healthy habits, like exercise and taking quiet time each day. Over the course of a year working together, Amanda lost twenty-five pounds and felt better than ever. Her A1C also fell into the normal range after some months, for which she was excited and thankful. Over time, she added a number of other approaches to help prevent recurrence, but losing weight was the one thing Amanda knew would optimize her health outcomes; she set the course, followed the recommendations, and found lasting success.

Nutritional Supplements

PERSONALLY, I REALLY like food. And as a naturopathic doctor, I like to think I could derive all the nourishment I need from the food and beverages I consume. I also appreciate that there is a role for nutritional supplements and that my patients who have been through conventional cancer care are universally interested in which, if any, supplements they should consider. Increasingly, supplements are being studied, either one by one or in combination, to better understand how they impact cells, tissue, organs, and people. Many supplements show the ability to help make conventional cancer care more effective, prevent side effects, address side effects that arise, help with "mopping up" post-treatment, improve quality of life, and help reduce the risk of recurrence.

A plethora of supplements are available online, in health food stores, in big-box stores, and in the kitchen cupboards and kitchen drawers of many households! I aim to streamline the decision-making for my patients and offer relevant recommendations, taking into consideration the type of cancer diagnosis, approaches taken, ongoing treatments, other underlying ailments, current symptoms, as well as cultural components and available resources.

That said, no one can—nor should they—take every supplement shown to have anticancer potential. First of all, it's cost-prohibitive. Secondly, it becomes cumbersome to take, say, ten pills, capsules, or powders numerous times a day. When I am with a patient, besides appreciating their health history, current medications, and health goals, I assess willingness, capacity, and interest in taking nutritional supplements, and then gear my prescriptions in such way as to match the person before me.

There are specific supplements for particular diagnoses, and others for symptoms that persist after cancer treatment. These are strictly individualized to the patient and vary widely. What is good for one person is not necessarily good for another. It is not reasonable to list out every narrowly prescribed supplement in this chapter. Please see chapter 17 for some more pointed recommendations based on common symptoms cancer survivors/thrivers experience.

I present here a compilation of broad-acting, anticancer supplements that are evidence-based and readily available. Note that all of the items listed also have other applications in health and wellness, but here I mainly share the information germane to cancer survivors.

✦ **CURCUMIN** (*Curcuma longa*), derived from the culinary herb turmeric, is at the top of most lists. It has been shown[85] to have both anti-inflammatory and anticancer attributes. Curcumin suppresses the initiation, progression, and metastasis of a number of cancer types. The mechanism of action seems to relate to both reducing angiogenesis (the creation of new blood vessels, which enable cancer cells to thrive) and interfering with tumor growth. Patients often ask me if they can get into a therapeutic range by using turmeric in their food. I would say it's wonderful and tasty to use in cooking, but if you are going for the anticancer impact, you want more than is palatable or realistic in a daily intake of food. Turmeric's positive impact is dose-dependent; in other words, more is better. I encourage patients to use the better-quality curcumin on the market.

✦ **GREEN TEA** (*Camellia sinensis*) and its principal constituent, EGCG (epigallocatechin gallate), should also be on your short list. It is a plant-based compound called a catechin, known for its strong antioxidant capacity. Antioxidants help sequester free radicals, which are the highly reactive particles that may cause damage in your cells. Many of the supplements suggested have an antioxidant effect. Green tea has been shown in numerous studies[86] to potentially decrease metastasis both *in vitro* (in laboratory studies) and *in vivo* (in people tested), and in epidemiological studies for some forms of cancer. Green tea appears to inhibit both tumor invasion and angiogenesis, essential for tumor growth and metastasis. You can drink green tea, mix it with other teas of your choice to enhance flavor, and find decaffeinated versions if you prefer. If you do not like the taste or want to amplify its therapeutic range, you can take green tea in supplement form.

✦ **MUSHROOMS** of many different varieties have been the focus of an enormous amount of research.[87] From one study,[88] we read, "The mounting evidences from various research groups across the globe regarding anti-tumor application of mushroom extracts unarguably make it a fast-track research area worth mass attention." I often prescribe a medical mushroom combination for my patients and also remind them to eat slightly sautéed mushrooms several times a week. When eaten raw, it is difficult to access the medicinal qualities due to the chitin layer, which makes up the cell wall in fungi. If overcooked, you destroy some of the pertinent anticancer components. Edible mushrooms like button mushrooms (*Agaricus bisporus*), oyster mushrooms (*Pleurotus ostreatus*), shiitake mushrooms (*Lentinus edodes*), and maitake mushrooms (*Grifola frondosa*) are worth including in the diet and will continue to be studied for their specific anticancer attributes. I have patients who just do not like mushrooms, so for them, powders derived from dried mushroom are a good alternative. And for everyone else, look for consistent intake of mushrooms perhaps two to three times a week.

✦ **QUERCETIN** is a flavonoid found in many fruits and vegetables. Flavonoids make up a range of phytonutrients, or plant chemicals, that give many of our fruits and vegetables their beautiful and appealing colors. The antioxidant capacity of flavonoids is both anti-inflammatory and immune system supporting. We find[89] an antiproliferative impact on a number of different cancer cell lines, *in vitro* and *in vivo*. This means it interferes with the reproduction and growth of cancer cells. Quercetin appears to support the process of *apoptosis*, or programmed destruction of cancer cells. Many people use quercetin for help during allergy season as well. It seems to stabilize mast cells, which release histamine, so it can reduce itchy eyes and watery noses caused by allergies.

✦ **MELATONIN** research[90] is burgeoning and gaining more and more study dollars. Melatonin appears to mitigate cancer both at the very beginning of the disease process and during progression. People have long used melatonin to help with insomnia, and indeed, when I recommend melatonin, I suggest patients take it before bed, not in the morning. Some patients report excessive dreaming with melatonin, in which case we work with lower doses.

✦ **RESVERATROL**, derived from grape skins, is antioxidant and pro-apoptotic. It has been studied especially with regard to colorectal and skin cancers,[91] but we can expect it would have general anticancer impact, and its side effect profile is nil.

✦ **ALPHA LIPOIC ACID** is another strong antioxidant that helps to stymy cancer cell proliferation. Research[92] supports its use as an anticancer agent.

✦ **VITAMIN D**, relevant for so many bodily functions, has a role to play in fighting back the development of cancer. Review studies[93] point to many of the mechanisms of action as well as the fact that vitamin D deficiency is a common and easily reversible issue.

✦ **FISH OIL** plays an enormous number of roles in biochemistry and health. Its anticancer capacity has been studied[94] for many types of cancer. Eating fish is also recommended.

✦ **PROBIOTICS** to help create a more robust microbiome are also suggested alongside fermented or cultured foods in the diet. A healthy microbiome supports proper digestion and nutrient absorption, a healthy immune system, and, as we increasingly understand, a better mood and clearer mind.

✦ **GARLIC AND GINGER** also show anticancer impact and can be taken in pill format. That said, I am a big fan of trying to take in as many of the anticancer items as possible as part of your diet. When I am making most any vegetable dish, I will start out sautéing onions and garlic, and add grated turmeric and ginger.

How much of which supplements to take and in what combination? This needs to be personalized to your current health status and other medical considerations, so I hope you will see a licensed naturopathic doctor or integrative medical provider who has expertise in these areas. Look for a provider who knows the pros and cons of the various approaches and is aware of drug/nutrient/supplement interactions.

There are clear contraindications for some supplements for some individuals and when taken in combination with other supplements or medications. For instance, if I have a patient who has a history of blood clot or stroke and is taking a blood thinner, I need to take special care with what supplement is prescribed and in what dosage, in order to prevent excessive bleeding. Supplements like vitamin C, curcumin, and fish oil are all mildly blood thinning.

My guiding tenet, as for all doctors, is "First, do no harm." Patients with cancer or who are now cancer-free want to be sure to find all the benefits from nutritional supplements and as few side effects as possible, so seeking the advice of a licensed naturopathic doctor or expert integrative doctor is essential.

It's also paramount to *eat food*, not just rely on supplements for your nutritional intake. There have been studies[95] showing that some cancer survivors err on the side of too many supplements and not enough healthy food, so I encourage my patients to think about their food intake *first* and dietary supplements *second*.

Patients often ask me *when* they should take their

supplements and if it should be with or without food. Recall that the fat-soluble vitamins A, D, E, and K need fat for optimal absorption. If you take a multivitamin, most contain those individual nutrients, so be sure there is some fat with the meal you are eating when you take those supplements. Supplements like fish oil, which is indicated for many people, and magnesium and iron, indicated for some, can each cause some stomach upset, so I generally recommend those be taken with meals as well. I discourage people from taking supplements right before bed, as your digestive system and absorption slow down then, so you do not receive the same benefit. The exception here would be melatonin, which can help you feel relaxed and bring on easier sleep, so it is not good to take melatonin during daytime hours.

I encourage my patients to find a pill box where they can lay out one to two weeks of supplements at a time, to make it easier and also to help them remember what they have taken. I like my patients to aim low and aim long, meaning to follow a manageable plan with consistency and success. If it's too overwhelming, you probably won't do it or stay with it, so it's good to employ any tools or tactics that can help!

Remember that nutritional supplements are just one part of a healing plan and need to be thought about in context of your overall health. Supplements and dosing should be reviewed every six months or so, or whenever there is a change in cancer status or any other acute or chronic ailment. As researchers continue to examine the role of nutritional supplements as they relate to cancer and to survivorship, we will continue to evolve how such substances are used in the clinical practice setting.

Patient Story

Leo came to me after being treated for melanoma. He brought in what can only be called an enormous box full of supplements he was taking. He had collected advice from friends, family members, the internet, and books he read. He was taking over 100 different supplements each day, which translated into even more nutrients and other substances as some of his products contained more than one item. He was overwhelmed and looking for a way to streamline his efforts. He wondered if any of them were doing any good. He had completed surgery and a course of chemotherapy and was now looking for ways to help reduce his potential for recurrence.

Leo also had high blood pressure and a strong family history of heart disease, so he wanted to include supplements that might help prevent or address those concerns.

I went to work trying to contextualize the melanoma as well as the hypertension into my overall understanding of Leo's health. We started first with recommendations around diet, exercise, and stress reduction, and then turned to the question of supplements. I was looking for those items with both anticancer and cardio-protective qualities. One aspect of nutritional supplements that I appreciate is that many have more than one indication, more than one way they can offer help. We started with fish oil, CoQ10, and vitamin D. I also suggested a multivitamin as he was working hard to move toward a healthier, anti-inflammatory diet but still struggled with fast food and too much alcohol. Over time we added further antioxidant nutritional supplements: alpha-lipoic acid and vitamin C. Leo was very happy to have a more streamlined set of supplements to add to his health plan without being overwhelmed by a cupboard full of pills. He also found he enjoyed his food more without constantly take a handful of pills before, during, or after his meals.

Botanical Medicine

I ADORE PLANTS. I adore the way they fill my home and my yard and other natural places, from city parks to natural landscapes where I enjoy spending time. I cherish bringing plant medicine to the clinic to help patients heal and stay healthy. Plants have been used as medicine since the earliest recorded history, in innumerable forms. Folk uses of medicinal plants are found everywhere from cave drawings to the Bible, and in languages circling the globe. Often it is the woman's purview, though not always, as knowledge and recipes are handed down the family tree.

Only in the last few decades have increased interest, resources, and scientific rigor been applied to the study of plant medicine. Particular botanicals I have prescribed for over thirty-six years now have some quality research explaining why and how they work.

For cancer patients and survivors, there are a growing number of herbs to consider. Many pharmaceuticals are *derived* from plants, including some cancer drugs like the vinca alkaloids (vinblastine, vincristine, and vindesine) and taxanes (paclitaxel and docetaxel).

Like drugs, there can be serious interactions between herbal remedies and other plants, medications, food, and supplements, so please seek guidance beyond "Dr. Google." Licensed naturopathic doctors have extensive training in botanical medicine, so if this is something you're interested in, find a local ND or certified herbalist for guidance to ensure appropriate prescribing and dosing for both efficacy and safety for you or your loved one.

We use some herbs to help *during* cancer care, such as to enhance the efficacy of chemotherapy, other drug treatments, or radiation, and also to help prevent or address side effects of treatment. Complaints I have helped patients with by prescribing herbs either during cancer care or afterwards for symptoms that persist include low blood counts, nausea, sad or anxious mood, sleep troubles, diarrhea, constipation, heart burn or gastroesophageal reflux, sore muscles, skin rashes, mouth sores, pain, brain fog, and more.

For people who have completed treatment, my main focus with botanical medicine is to first "mop up" any persistent side effects from care. I want to help my patients feel restored in particular areas that are often hardest hit, as in the list above, while individualizing recommendations to each patient. See chapter 17 to see how botanicals fit into patient plans for specific post-treatment complaints.

We also use botanicals to help reduce the risk of further cancer. Many substances derived from the plant world show anticancer activity and carry low side-effect profiles. I rarely prescribe herbs as stand-alone treatment, as the collective chapters of this book reflect. Instead, I contextualize and individualize botanical medicine offerings within the overall plan for my patient, which includes dietary encouragement, the exercise prescription, attention to the patient's emotional world, and other integrative medicine tools. That said, herbal medicine is a cornerstone of patient care for many licensed naturopathic doctors, myself included.

I have particular affinity for recommending culinary herbs, which are often readily available, affordable, and used widely. For other plant medicines, I may suggest they be taken as a tea or as a tincture extract, or in capsule form. I like working with whole herbs rather than isolated herbal components for the elements that are less definable or extractable in the lab but may nonetheless be in play and beneficial. However, some of my patients prefer botanicals in a supplement-like format, with compressed pills or encapsulated, freeze-dried, desiccated material, where active ingredients are measured and standardized.

I take into consideration cultural norms, budget, and capacity for consistency when suggesting which herbs to take, in what preparation, and how often. The generally anticancer herbs I use with cancer survivors include the following:

✦ **FOR THE CULINARY HERBS, MY FAVORITE GO-TO TRIO** is garlic[96] (*Allium sativa*), turmeric[97] (*Curcuma longa*), and ginger[98] (*Zingiber officinale*). Each has been studied and shows anticancer impact. I encourage patients to use these herbs liberally in cooking—such as pressing garlic and grating ginger root and turmeric root into warm oil to begin a stir-fry. Both ginger root and turmeric root freeze well, last a very long time, and are easy to grate directly from the freezer. When you're preparing your cooked vegetable and protein dishes, start with any and all of these three easy-to-find botanicals.

✦ **IT'S WORTH REPEATING THAT MUSHROOMS,** as described in chapter 7, show[99] tremendous promise against cancer and can be eaten as food and/or taken in pill form. When eaten they should be slightly steamed or sautéed because it's difficult to access the medicinal qualities of raw mushrooms due to the chitin, or outer cell-wall layers. But if overcooked, less of the active components remain. Dried mushrooms retain much of their medicinal qualities and are considerably more affordable. Soak in water for a few minutes before including in a stir-fry or other cooked dishes. Other types of mushrooms less typically found in the grocery produce department have been shown to be especially cancer-preventing, and often I prescribe these in capsules or powdered form.

✦ **BERBERINE OFFICINALIS,** derived from Oregon grape and other plants, is shown[100] to be cytotoxic (cell killing) to cancer cells and to inhibit cell proliferation or the making of more cells. It also helps regulate blood sugar by enhancing insulin sensitivity. This helps to down-regulate certain inflammatory pathways, which has anticancer benefits.

✦ **ASTRAGALUS MEMBRANACEUS** is a powerhouse botanical studied[101] for its impact on cell proliferation and apoptosis, or encouraging natural cell death to cancer cells. It also helps enhance immunity and balance stress hormones so is often on my recommended short list. In chapter 11, I focus on the negative impact of incessant stress. For many people, especially cancer survivors, stress is ever present. *Astragalus* is an herb for our time.

✦ **GREEN TEA (CAMELLIA SINENSIS)** preparations, by the cup or taken in pill fashion, caffeinated or not, show clear evidence[102] of reducing the risk of cancer. For those who do not care for the taste, it's fine to combine green tea with other preferred flavored herbal teas or diluted fruit juices.

✦ **RESVERATROL**, derived from the skin of red grapes, blueberries, raspberries, and mulberries, is also described in chapter 7. Resveratrol is a strong antioxidant that has been shown[103] to slow cancer cellular proliferation.

✦ **GINSENG (PANAX GINSENG)** is a star when examined[104] in both the laboratory and in people, showing a positive effect in preventing cancer. Ginseng works in many ways to inhibit tumor formation, support apoptosis, inhibit angiogenesis, and more.

Just as important, it's essential to know which botanicals *not* to use! For those who had a blood cancer, we are careful *not* to prescribe botanicals that stimulate immune function, such as *Echinaceae*, *Astragalus*, or the mushrooms described above. There are other herbs in this category as well, which underscores the importance of securing professional advice before creating a plan that includes botanical medicine.

And then, because many patients had or continue to have other illnesses beyond cancer, I sometimes recommend an herbal preparation to help with specific concerns. In some instances, this allows a patient to avoid, reduce, or discontinue a pharmaceutical. While this is not the goal of naturopathic medicine, if I can assist a patient to take one less drug, if indicated, I do. The phenomenon of the prescribing cascade, where one drug is given and causes symptoms that require another drug, is sadly a common occurrence. Polypharmacy presents its own issues, so I am mindful of all the medications my patients take and offer information about other approaches, including botanical medicine, where we might be able to lower dosage or discontinue a medication. I do this in communication with the prescribing physician. To read more about deprescribing, see chapter 10.

Here are a few good examples of using botanicals with survivors who have other kinds of concerns:

Patients with gastroesophageal reflux (GERD) are often prescribed drugs like Zantac or proton pump inhibitors (PPIs), which have serious potential side effects[105] when taken in the long term. These patients often do well with licorice root[106] (*Glycyrrhiza glabra*), which soothes the mucous membrane lining of the esophagus. I might also add in slippery elm (*Ulmus fulva*) lozenges, which also help. Studies[107] show that potable aloe vera juice, if you don't mind the slime factor, offers relief. We can use these on a regular basis as a preventive and also for occasional GERD symptoms. It's important to note that research is showing that PPIs, one of the most commonly prescribed medications, put people at increased risk for osteoporosis[108]; kidney, liver, and cardiovascular disease; dementia; respiratory and digestive infections; and impaired absorption of nutrients.[109]

For those struggling with sleep I offer lavender (*Lavandula*)[110] in all its many forms. An added benefit[111] is that it may also lead to improvement in depression and anxiety. Huge swaths of patients have become addicted to benzodiazepines when searching for better sleep, and people have a hard time quitting. Herbal medicine used within a whole-person, natural medicine approach can help with benzodiazepine withdrawal and can also help address underlying causes of insomnia. Review chapter 12 for more specific information and help with sleep troubles.

For garden-variety illnesses such as sore throat, slippery elm (*Ulmus fulva*) can help. Elderberry (*Sambucus nigra*) in its various forms has shown efficacy[112] in the prevention and treatment of flu and upper respiratory infection.

There are many other complaints you might have. Regardless of what part of the body is hurting and based on how you experience your symptoms, there is often an herbal medicine to consider. See chapter 17 for more thoughts on using botanical medicines aimed at common complaints that arise or remain after cancer care.

While you are working to create a plan for health and vitality, remember the power of herbs. Seek advice from a knowledgeable person who has experience working with cancer survivors. Be sure to share all other supplements and medications you are taking, to prevent unwanted interactions. And the next time you're out and about, enjoying the living plants around you, give a small nod to the role they play in our daily lives and in the healing medicine cabinet.

Patient Story

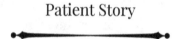

When Maura completed care for estrogen receptor–positive breast cancer, she was prescribed tamoxifen. Though she knew it was the right medicine for her, she struggled with side effects of joint pain, or arthralgia. It interfered with her desire and capacity for exercise, which she knew was a key part of her recovery from cancer care and staying healthy. She also reported that her range of motion, especially in her arms, was compromised. She did not have lymphedema or peripheral neuropathy.

She came to me for help for the side effects from the medication. Though I am a doctor who prioritizes addressing the root cause, in Maura's case, I knew that the risk–benefit related to long-term use of tamoxifen made it clear she should remain on this medication if at all possible.

In my experience with hormone-blocking medications, both for women and for men, one component of the side effects relates to underlying tendencies that person may already have. This is not universally true, but clinically, I often see this. Some people have an initial challenge with the medication but eventually adapt. It had been about eight months since Maura began tamoxifen, and she felt she was getting progressively worse. Her oncologist recommended anti-inflammatory medication, which she did not want to take.

Maura was already eating an anti-inflammatory diet and had removed a number of foods to which she was sensitive. She was also taking fish oil. I recommended the botanical medicines *Boswellia serrata*,[113] known for its anti-inflammatory capacity, alongside curcumin (*Curcuma longa*),[114] a tried-and-true herb to help reduce inflammation and swelling, among its many other roles.

After a month with these botanicals, Maura returned to the office very pleased. Her pain levels were greatly reduced, and she felt like she had a more normal range of motion. She continued to use these herbs over the years spanning her tamoxifen treatment and then discontinued them slowly when her antiestrogen treatments were complete.

Whole-Person Medicines:
Homeopathy/Acupuncture

ACUPUNCTURE AND HOMEOPATHY are *whole-person* approaches to health, and I recommend them for a number of reasons to cancer survivors or those currently in treatment. "Mopping up" from conventional care is high on that list. Surgery, chemotherapy, radiation, and other approaches are hard on the body, and these whole-person approaches can help patients recover and regain health and vitality.

Addressing everyday illnesses that come up—preventing them or treating them naturally—is another goal. Pharmaceutical prescriptions are often offered for these ailments, but the more drugs we add to a prescription list, the more potential side effects we encounter. Gentle natural medicines, including whole-person approaches, often provide adequate help by working to stimulate your inherent healing capacity.

Addressing other underlying chronic disease is important, too, because for many people, cancer is *only one* of a number of serious or concerning diagnoses. Quality of life is often impacted by other chronic ailments, so using whole-person approaches can channel healing potential toward helping reverse or slow the impact of concurrent diseases.

Offering help with general symptoms such as fatigue, anxiety, depression, insomnia, and an overall lack of well-being is something we can accomplish with whole-person approaches alongside therapeutic nutrition, botanical medicine, exercise, and working on the head game, as described in other chapters of this book.

Here I would like to discuss acupuncture and homeopathy and how they each offer effective, evidence-informed approaches to support and stimulate the body's inherent healing capacity to address both acute and chronic complaints. We know we are more than the sum of our parts, yet medicine, including natural medicine, often breaks us down to all the component pieces. Sometimes this is essential and quite effective, but a broader holistic approach is also relevant. Although acupuncture and homeopathy are vastly different areas of study, research, and application, they are both overarching, organizing systems of the human body. We can identify these systems and how they may not be working effectively, and then work to correct those imbalances. By stimulating the body's inherent healing capacity, these gentle approaches help patients reach a more balanced and healthier state.

In this chapter, I will not offer specific homeopathic remedies or acupuncture plans to utilize—because these treatments are by definition *entirely* individualized to a patient at a moment in time. But let's take these four areas for potential help and support listed above and discuss them a little further: "mopping up," treating acute illness, treating chronic disease, and helping with overall sense of well-being.

✦   **"MOPPING UP."** Surgery and other procedures, radiation and chemotherapy, and other cancer treatments are strong and intense for good reason; they each have an enormous job to do. And for some, medication or treatments are overlapping and/or continuing. We can use homeopathy or acupuncture to help address symptoms that remain or bothersome side effects due to conventional cancer care.

✦ **TREATING ACUTE DISEASE.** As a cancer survivor and thriver, or as someone living with cancer, sometimes you suffer an injury or are what I like to call "normal sick." It's part of being alive—from colds and sore throats to bruises and sprained ankles. With cancer survivors, I am more aware of how I work to *prevent* acute ailments and especially how I treat them, because I want to help patients focus on the bigger picture. I want my patients to avoid other drugs if possible. I want to help the body heal itself from these kinds of problems. The human body is beautifully equipped to handle quite a number of illnesses and injuries when given the right ingredients, appropriate support, and time for healing. Homeopathy and acupuncture shine in this realm.

With acute illnesses where the immune system is working to fight an infection, research[115] on homeopathy shows positive impact. Other patient studies[116] reflect homeopathy's efficacy in treating cough and bronchitis. If we can use homeopathy for acute illness and help patients side-step antibiotics, it's a good idea. Antibiotics are life-saving but also terribly overprescribed, leading to a pending worldwide emergency[117] of antibiotic-resistant infections. Taking antibiotics also reduces the diversity and robustness of your microbiome, which negatively impacts your immune system. Homeopathy is shown to be effective when single specific remedies are individualized for your particular symptoms of an acute illness.

I value homeopathy because at its core, it's both holistic

and *vitalistic*. Vitalism is the idea that as living organisms, we are more than our biochemical reactions alone. Many of us found naturopathic or integrative medicine because we were drawn by the ideas of holism and vitalism, yet our tools are increasingly reductionist, focused on minutiae of specific biochemical reactions—in a word, *mechanistic*. Not that such tools are unimportant or do not work, and believe me, as a cancer survivor/thriver myself, I employ many of them myself *and* with my patients! But when I can use or refer a patient for a whole-person medicine like homeopathy or acupuncture, I welcome the opportunity and outcomes.

I also draw tremendous satisfaction and see positive clinical results when I can look at my patient as a whole person and select a homeopathic medicine that addresses their physical, cognitive, and emotional aspects. Homeopathy stimulates the patient's innate healing ability, and this is in sync with how I understand people, nature, and healing. Lastly, the homeopathic interview, the process of gathering information to make a prescription, is itself healing for both doctor and patient. For the doctor because it allows us to connect with our patient in loving and meaningful ways, and for the patient, who in turn feels heard and supported.

In a review article,[118] acupuncture treatment showed promise for "pain . . . including its use in chemotherapy-induced peripheral neuropathy, aromatase inhibitor-associated arthralgia, post neck dissection pain," and more. In another meta-analysis,[119] acupuncture significantly lowered many treatment-related symptoms in survivors and is known to have a very low side-effect profile. Based on the data examined, researchers recommend acupuncture be added to cancer care symptom management.

The experience of receiving acupuncture for many people is relaxing and soothing. There is hands-on touch, there is the taking of pulses at the wrist, the assessment of the tongue, and, overall, a more holistic assessment of the person. While the therapy itself is shown to be effective for specific complaints, I never underestimate the value for a patient of being seen as a whole person, allowing someone else to engage with direct healing and work to stimulate the body's inherent capacity for balance and health.

✦ **ADDRESSING UNDERLYING CHRONIC DISEASE.** I am also interested in addressing other underlying chronic diseases for a number of reasons. Some ailments put people at risk for further cancer. I would hate to be part of helping you beat cancer while meanwhile you fall ill or suffer from another, largely lifestyle-related and preventable ailment like heart disease or diabetes. I would put chronic psycho-emotional ailments here, too, as the mind affects the nervous system, the nervous system impacts the immune system, and round and round we go. In a review study,[120] positive results were observed from the use of homeopathy in chronic disease. Chronic pain belongs in this category, suffered by many people with and without cancer. In a meta-analysis,[121] acupuncture was shown to be effective for the treatment of chronic pain, and the improvements persisted over time.

✦ **GENERAL WELL-BEING.** The last category might be the most important. What do we mean by a general sense of well-being? For many cancer survivors, it means relaxing again, getting back to life with some semblance of normalcy. It means not always thinking or worrying about cancer. For others, it means getting back to work or returning to family responsibilities, hobbies, travel, volunteer efforts, creative pursuits, and more.

With homeopathy, we can impact general well-being by prescribing a remedy for the whole person, not their diagnosis; we call this a constitutional remedy. We individualize the prescription based on how the person experiences their symptoms and also factoring in their temperament, personality, general physical tendencies, energy level, and more. A constitutional homeopathic remedy can have a positive impact on self-agency, mental clarity, and vitality while also addressing specific physical body symptoms.

Similarly, acupuncture can be used to improve the overall health and well-being of a patient, not only to provide symptomatic relief. There is increasing evidence[122] that supports acupuncture's ability to help the whole person in this way.

Another whole-person approach with centuries of use from the Indian tradition is called Ayurvedic medicine. Ayurveda focuses on preventive care and treating with lifestyle approaches like massage, mindfulness, yoga, botanical medicines, and specific diet based on body and humoral type. There is a complicated if elegant philosophy to Ayurveda, and over time, I imagine that Ayurvedic approaches will be more rigorously studied and show relevance for whole-person health.

I like to offer patients choices in the therapies they consider, because some approaches work better for some people than others. Also, having options is empowering. When you've improved your habits and made lifestyle changes to regain your health or to live with cancer as best you can, but you feel you need a little more help and support, consider adding homeopathy and/or acupuncture to your efforts. Look for an experienced, credentialed provider, whether through word of mouth or a credentialing agency. And recall that health care is deeply personal and that no one kind of approach has all the answers. Putting together your dream team of providers might take time, but using different perspectives and integrating your care often offers the best results. As indicated, including acupuncture and homeopathy as part of a treatment plan will be a fine complement to other approaches.

Patient Stories

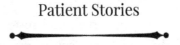

Alicia, age forty-five, came to see me six months after finishing treatment for early breast cancer. She'd had a lumpectomy and radiation on her left side, which caused lymphedema in her left arm. She was also suffering with a full-body rash that was red, slightly raised, and itchy. The rash was worse when she became warm, especially after a shower, while in bed, or if she began to perspire when walking. Alicia came from an impressive line of long-lived people and had taken good care of herself. Except for the breast cancer, she let me know she was quite healthy. She also had a great attitude, telling me, "Look, bad things happen to good people," and she was just going to "get on with it" and do what she could to live a healthy, long life and to enjoy her family.

Based on her symptoms, temperament, and health history, I prescribed the homeopathic remedy *Sulphur* to address her specific complaints and to support her overall health. I also instructed Alicia on how to use hydrotherapy at home to help with the lymphedema. (See chapter 13 for more on hydrotherapy, and see the section on lymphedema in chapter 17.) I also advised her about eating anti-inflammatory foods and bringing more relaxation into her busy life.

When Alicia returned to see me one month later, the swelling and range of motion in her arm were much improved. "I'm feeling good again!" she told me excitedly. The rash, while still visible, was fading and no longer itchy. Over the next couple of months, Alicia's rash disappeared, and her lymphedema was barely noticeable. Alicia was pleased and has continued to see me off and on, as needed, for the past ten years. She has remained cancer-free, for which she is deeply grateful.

Not every patient with lymphedema will respond to the remedy *Sulphur*. There are many other remedies I have found helpful for my post-cancer patients, who present with a wide range of symptoms, varying levels of overall health, and unique personalities and temperaments—all of which need to be taken into account when prescribing a homeopathic remedy tailored to the individual. That's why it is essential to seek personalized care from a credentialed homeopathic practitioner.

I reached out to a colleague and friend, Bonnie Diamond, MAc, a licensed acupuncturist in Easthampton, Massachusetts, to see if she might share a survivor patient story. Keep in mind that some of the things Bonnie describes may seem far-fetched. But acupuncture has a very long history and all kinds of research to support its efficacy. Sometimes things that seem foreign or strange are just new to us. I try to keep an open mind!

From Bonnie:

Bob, a sixty-two-year-old man, came to see me four years ago to find relief from left-sided shoulder pain. The pain had started six months earlier and had gotten progressively worse. At age fifty-four, Bob had been treated for throat cancer. He received radiation, chemotherapy, and had a temporary feeding tube placed. Bob seemed to enjoy life and was extremely grateful to receive the cancer treatment he needed. He was taking medication to control his blood pressure, but was otherwise healthy.

I practice a Japanese style of acupuncture based on the work of world-renowned acupuncturist Kiiko Matsumoto. In this style, we palpate the body to find restrictions and release those restrictions with needles, magnets, and electrical stimulation.

The only restriction I could find on palpation was on the back left side of Bob's neck. I used acupuncture needles according to guidelines to release this area. I added another potent point for neck pain, and points along the stomach meridian that smooth out the pulse.

During the second part of the treatment, I inserted three needles around the tight shoulder area and attached triple bypass cords, which direct the flow of ions in and around cells where there is pain and inflammation. I used a battery-operated device that emitted small static electrical sparks. This treatment is based on the work of Japanese master Kawaii.

I sent Bob home with 800-gauss magnets taped onto the left shoulder area. By the end of the second treatment, Bob was feeling enormous relief, and after five visits the pain was completely gone.

Four years later, Bob returned. His left shoulder was fine, but he now had pain on his right side. He came back for four visits. I started with the same treatment. After two visits, the pain had diminished slightly, but the change was not as dramatic as when he first came to see me. I added a muscle-relaxing treatment at that time. Then I applied a traditional Chinese medicine technique called gua sha, which can be translated to "scraping the wind." I used a porcelain Chinese soup spoon to scrape the shoulder area after covering it with coconut oil. By the fourth visit Bob's pain was completely gone. For patients that have symptoms remaining after cancer care, acupuncture and Chinese medicine have much to offer.

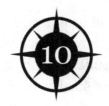

Using Prescribed Medication Alongside Natural Medicine and the Off-Label Use of Pharmaceuticals

AS A LICENSED naturopathic doctor, I rely first on natural medicine approaches for preventing and treating illness. However, I also advocate for the appropriate, judicious use of prescription medication. NDs are trained to prescribe pharmaceutical agents according to the standard of care.

For better or worse, for cancer survivors and everyone else, we have become a nation of pill lovers. A 2019 report shows[123] that 69 percent of adults aged forty to seventy-nine take at least one prescription drug, and 24 percent take over five prescriptions. This leads to a whole challenge of polypharmacy, the use of more than one drug at a time. The more drugs someone takes, the more chance for side effects to develop and drug interactions to occur. Adverse events due to overprescribing are especially likely for our oldest adults, who metabolize medications more slowly and differently than younger people and who are, sadly, often overtreated.

In 1991, geriatrician Mark H. Beers created the Beers Criteria for Potentially Inappropriate Medication Use in Older Adults.[124] This evidence-based resource,[125] updated every three years, is an essential tool for all health-care professionals who treat older patients. Applying its recommendations supports the safer prescribing of pharmaceuticals for the geriatric set.

Because children are smaller in size and also metabolize medications differently, their prescriptions require special attention too. An important resource[126] is the KIDS List (Key Potentially Inappropriate Drugs in Pediatrics) to educate, inform, and offer essential information for practitioners about commonly prescribed drugs for kids.

These resources include information on the concept of deprescribing to help reduce issues that arise from drug-drug interaction and adverse effects. Sometimes that means reducing doses, as side effects are often dose-dependent. It may also mean working toward complete elimination of a drug in question. There are also useful apps with similar information. The topic of deprescribing has been increasingly studied[127] as more physicians become aware of polypharmacy pitfalls and work to minimize unneeded medications.

Some of my patients come into my office with the express desire to get off certain medications, but I do not always support these goals. All medicine needs to be individualized and personalized to the patient. Many medications for cancer survivors are prescribed to prevent further cancer or recurrence, and I generally recommend those be continued.

In fact, when research supports the efficacy of such approaches, but the patient is reluctant or has challenging side effects, I encourage the patient to remain on the drug. We work together to reverse or address side effects. This is especially true for hormonal treatments, immunotherapies, and targeted therapies. I draw from my naturopathic tool kit to address symptoms and see if we can reap the benefits of the medication with few or fewer side effects. If a patient is reluctant for more philosophical reasons, I will share the research, the statistics, and any other information so the patient can best understand their options.

You may be taking drugs for other non-cancer-related diagnoses. The vast majority of chronic illnesses for which drugs are prescribed are lifestyle and natural medicine preventable or treatable. Among the most commonly prescribed medications in this country are drugs for chronic pain, hypothyroidism, high cholesterol, hypertension, type 2 diabetes, and gastroesophageal reflux. You will find effective natural and integrative medicine recommendations for many of these diagnoses, and others, when you work with a naturopathic or integrative medical doctor. The public-facing Institute for Natural Medicine website[128] maintains a robust resource section that shares research, information, and clinical pearls, free of charge, for many of these illnesses and others. For complaints specific to people who have been through cancer care, such as fatigue, brain fog, lymphedema, peripheral neuropathy, and sexual concerns, please refer to chapter 17.

It's important to note that certain commonly prescribed medications may interfere with therapies aimed at cancer prevention. For example, selective serotonin reuptake inhibitors (SSRIs), a category of antidepressants, inhibit an enzyme that may slow the metabolism of the anticancer drug tamoxifen,[129] possibly decreasing its efficacy. Other commonly used drugs that may interfere with tamoxifen metabolism include quinidine, used for abnormal heart rhythm; certain antihistamines; and cimetidine, used to lower stomach acid. If you are taking tamoxifen alongside one of these drugs, you should not stop taking the medication, but please discuss this research with your prescribing physician, and also consider other natural medicine approaches to address the complaints that led to those prescriptions.

Many life-saving medications, from hormone blockers to immunotherapies, have a long list of potential side effects. You can be proactive when you know these risks. For instance, hormone-blocking drugs increase possibility of bone density loss. This makes weight-bearing exercise and resistance training that much more important, alongside adequate intake of foods high in calcium, vitamin D, and vitamin K, and possibly supplementation. It is imperative to seek support and be proactive to help prevent such common side effects.

Immunotherapy is often a mainstay of cancer treatment, and may be taken for years. While many people tolerate immunotherapy well, the list of potential side effects is long, including skin reactions, flu-like feelings, hormonal changes, headaches, shortness of breath, edema, and more. Consider working with a provider who can assist with natural medicine approaches tailored to your side effects and which will not interfere with immunotherapy efficacy so that you can stay on a potentially life-saving immuno-targeted therapy regimen.

Other kinds of targeted therapies, like PARP inhibitors, are showing tremendous promise for treating some cancers and preventing spread of disease. Poly adenosine diphosphate-ribose polymerase (PARP) is an enzyme that helps repair DNA damage in cells. PARP *inhibitors* work hard to prevent cancer cells from repairing, which ultimately allows those cells to die. PARP inhibitors, initially prescribed after chemotherapy, are now being used and studied earlier in treatment for metastatic breast, pancreatic, and ovarian cancers, as well as others. Common side effects include headache, vertigo, and hypertension, though these medications have largely been proven safe. Addressing such side effects with natural medicine approaches can help a person stay on an otherwise helpful medication.

As I work over weeks and months with patients to address their complaints, there may come a time when we consider reducing the dose or deprescribing a drug if it no longer seems relevant. We do this in communication with the prescribing physician.

Off-Label Use of Pharmaceuticals

There is increasing evidence that off-label use of certain medications may provide help in prevention and treatment of cancer and the prevention of recurrence. The concept of drug repurposing is not new. Beyond the evidence of efficacy are economic reasons to consider drug repositioning. Statistics[130] show that from 2006 to 2015, about 12 percent of drugs went from phase 1 trial to FDA approval. For oncology drugs, the number hovered at just 5 percent.

This means that there are not that many new drugs coming to market for any particular cancer in any particular year. The incidence of cancer and difficult-to-treat cancers is outpacing the rate at which new drugs are approved. As the occurrence of cancer across the globe increases, access to expensive cancer drugs remains a challenge. Researchers are working[131] to articulate characteristics in non-cancer drugs to study in order to figure out which medications show the most promise in oncology.

In general, ideal drugs would be readily available, affordable, carry low side-effect profiles, and have the clincher attributes: the capacity to prevent cancer and/or to slow the growth and spread of cancer cells. In addition, they should have a history of use, hopefully for many years, reflecting both safety and tolerability. Many of these repurposed drugs are also studied to be used *simultaneously* during conventional cancer care, to make cancer cells more radio-sensitive, chemo-sensitive, or medication-sensitive. Whether an off-label use of a non-cancer drug is relevant during or after cancer care is a topic to discuss with your medical provider.

Some of the drugs considered and studied came to light because of statistical analyses. The best example here is metformin. Studies[132] show that cancer patients with diabetes who take metformin have considerably better outcomes. Metformin, used by many prediabetic and diabetic patients to keep blood sugar in the normal range, is derived from the plant *Galega officinalis* and has been used for over fifty years. Because of this long history, we know it's generally safe. Many clinical trials[133] underway are looking into the role metformin may play in both the prevention and treatment of cancer.

Metformin lowers blood sugar in several ways, including decreasing the amount of sugar absorbed from the digestive tract, reducing the overall amount of sugar made by the liver, and raising insulin sensitivity. Metformin inhibits other biochemical pathways, which in turn helps slow tumor growth. Research[134] also shows that metformin helps address cancer stem cells and seems to stop precancerous cells from changing into cancerous ones. The hardest part of taking metformin may be convincing your provider to prescribe it for you if you are not prediabetic or diabetic.

On a related note: the botanical medicine berberine (*Berberis vulgaris*) has long been used to treat diarrhea, but it is increasingly appreciated[135] for the many metabolic pathways it impacts, including those related to blood sugar regulation (see chapter 8). So some of my patients who want the blood sugar support of metformin but do not want to take another medication opt for taking supplemental berberine. Berberine, however, is considerably more expensive than the generic form of metformin.

Proton pump inhibitors (PPIs), commonly taken to reduce stomach acid, are another class of medications being considered[136] for possible anticancer impact. There are proton pumps within tumor cells that have similar characteristics to those in the stomach. The hypothesis is that blocking those with PPIs may make chemotherapy and immune therapies work better by lowering the acid level in the tumor environment. That said, PPIs, especially when used in the long term, are associated with increased risk of certain cancers, so weighing the risk-benefit is complicated. And, as described elsewhere, other complications can occur with regular use of PPIs.

Common aspirin is an over-the-counter medication sometimes used after cancer treatment. Data[137] suggests that daily low-dose aspirin is associated with a reduction in all-cause mortality (death) in cancer survivors. Care should be taken with use of other medications that are blood thinning or supplements that have mild blood-thinning potential, such as fish oil, bromelain, curcumin, and vitamin C.

To be clear, many repurposed medications are not aimed at specific kinds of cancers or cancer cells. Instead, they aim at the microenvironment where cancer cells develop and grow. The upside of repurposed medication is, again, that issues around dosing and common side effects, if they exist, are often already known. And most are readily available and inexpensive. There are growing lists and studies being created to dive deeper into this field. One clearing house keeps a database[138] of drugs considered.

Hundreds of research studies[139] show efficacy of specific non-cancer drugs, depending on cancer type, patient history, and more. The list includes many well-known drugs you have heard of, from chloroquine to beta blockers to lithium to Simvastatin. If you have completed cancer care, consider having a conversation with your oncologist about other known medications that might be of potential benefit in your care. Or at the very least, if you are on a medication for a certain illness, see if there are other medications in that class of drugs that may also carry some anticancer capacity.

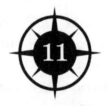

The Head Game, Stress, and Stress Reduction

STRONG EMOTIONS DURING and after cancer treatment are extremely common—while also worrying about, in no particular order, your health, your livelihood, your relationships, your sex life, your family, and your very mortality! What approaches, skills, and attitudes can help you manage stress and raise your threshold for feeling stress? What tools can support your ability to experience a wide range of emotions but not become stuck in any one of them? There are many, and I put them in a category I call the head game.

A cancer diagnosis can be a huge blow. The shock, the details of complicated decision-making, and the treatment process itself can bring on emotional and physical stress. Post-treatment time may present a host of other stressful situations, decision-making, and overwhelm. As you rejoin society and social circles, you may face unexpected challenges. Work may provide a positive or negative setting, or your family dynamics may have shifted. Once treatment is completed, you may experience a potent mix of exhilaration, anxiety, fear, depression, overwhelm, terror, anger, and relief.

All those emotions are normal and part of life, and they need to be given time and attention. In the book *Burnout: The Secret to Unlocking the Stress Cycle*,[140] Emily and Amelia Nagoski beautifully describe the neurobiology of the stress cycle. They write about how every emotion has a beginning, a middle, and an end. You have to feel your emotion and get all the way through it in order to move on. When feelings come back around, you will again have to feel your feelings to help you move past them.

The authors suggest, and I concur entirely, that there are many ways to process emotions, including talking about them, having a good cry, doing deep breathing, sharing a caring hug, having a deep belly laugh, doing something creative like writing, drawing, or singing, and feeling connected to and supported by family and friends. Feeling emotions thoroughly, especially the more challenging ones, is an important part of moving forward.

With patients in my practice, I encourage exploring all kinds of skills, tools, and practices to help with the head game. I allow time during our office visit to talk about feelings and to make space for this essential and evolving part of the healing process. I like to focus on habits people can create to raise their threshold for feeling stress and to move through the stress response. Then, if problems persist, I often prescribe an individualized treatment plan that includes specific natural medicine prescriptions, especially to help keep the twin feelings of anxiety and depression at bay.

There is a Japanese word, *kintsugi*, which refers to a 500-year-old technique of using gold to repair broken pottery. This makes the repaired cracks very visible, highlighting them rather than hiding them, thereby writing something notable into the object's history. Similarly, after cancer treatment, we may not go back to exactly how we were before, but we can create a "new normal" that also works, hopefully has some perks, and allows us to get back to life and continue to evolve. Much of this depends on a strong and consistent head game.

You may have a long, complex relationship with anxiety, depression, irritability, and other psycho-emotional challenges. Or you may have been blessed with a sturdy emotional life, guided by a positive outlook, and filled with examples of emotional agility, optimism, and resilience. Regardless of where you started, anxiety and depression related to having cancer, completing treatment, or living with cancer are almost universal. Some chemotherapeutic agents even have depression as a *known* side effect. In this case, the benefit—addressing the cancer—outweighs the risk, but nonetheless, you may be left with challenging feelings that interfere with being at peace and enjoying your life.

Conventional cancer treatments—surgery, chemotherapy, and radiation—are notorious for creating biological mechanisms that lead to inflammation,[141] which in turn, through a number of biochemical pathways, may further lead to the psycho-emotional symptoms.

Patients ask me why stress has such a strong impact on their physical and emotional health. With unrelenting stress,[142] the *sympathetic* nervous system is *stimulated*, which causes fast and involuntary responses to uncomfortable, stressful, or scary situations. You may feel your heart race, or your thoughts jumble. You may have an upset stomach or feel dizzy. When stress is continuous, this response does not have a chance to entirely subside.

Likewise, with unrelenting stress and worry, *inhibition* of the *parasympathetic* nervous system negatively affects your capacity for rest, sleep, and digestion. The parasympathetic response helps to decrease respiration and heart rate and also supports effective digestion. The combination of a jacked-up sympathetic nervous system and an ineffective parasympathetic response leads many people to feel anxious, depressed, and/or irritable. You are not alone if you feel stressed out; there are biochemical and hormonal reactions taking place that cause those uncomfortable feelings.

The long arm of unabated stress also activates the brain's

hypothalamus, the pituitary gland, and the adrenal glands, which in optimal health work in harmony. But when this hormonal axis is continually stressed, for some people it will lead to longer-lasting depression and anxiety.

Fear of cancer recurrence in particular often leads to excessive bodily awareness, where you interpret sensations that are not particularly relevant to disease as symptoms of cancer pathology, a phenomenon known as *somatosensory amplification*. From my own experience, this can occasionally veer toward humor. For instance, I once accidently hit my head pretty hard on a doorframe. The next day I had a bruise on my forehead and a headache. Hard to believe, but I briefly thought and blurted out, "I hope I don't have brain cancer." My husband looked at me, eyes widening, and we both started laughing. Clearly, this was so far from reasonable, even absurd, but I imagine you have had similar experiences.

Depression[143] decreases quality of life, increases physical symptoms, and, not surprisingly, negatively impacts families. In cancer patients, depression increases hospital stays, dollars spent, and the risk of suicide. And a cancer diagnosis followed by treatment is psycho-emotionally challenging for most every patient. The more these ideas are studied, the more we learn that cultivating an upbeat outlook and using skills to keep anxiety and depression at bay make a difference. Research[144] underscores that depression and anxiety have a negative effect on quality of life, of course, *but also on actual health outcomes and survival*. Mood impacts immune function, which impacts disease progression and mortality.

I want you to appreciate that adopting and committing to improving your head game is a worthwhile pursuit because *you can change* the biochemistry related to your stress response. Some of us are hardwired for mental health challenges, through our genes, our upbringing, and our previous life experiences. But change is always possible. It's never too late to take on qualities and skills that can shift your perspective and help ease psychological challenges. Keep reading for ways to help yourself. And know that there are natural medicine approaches to help when your symptoms are too much to bear.

Let's first address the medications often offered. For some, these are life-saving, and the benefits outweigh the risks. For others, not so much.

Pharmaceuticals such as SSRIs (e.g., Prozac, Lexapro) and benzodiazepines (e.g., Xanax, Ativan) are commonly prescribed to patients suffering emotionally. Sometimes this is due to doctor recommendation, and sometimes patients ask for a medication by name. One meta-analysis[145] found no advantage among drugs given. Some SSRIs can worsen[146] nausea and vomiting *during* treatment. And SSRIs have been shown[147] to decrease the time to disease progression in ovarian cancer patients. SSRIs also may interfere with efficacy of some estrogen-blocking medications, which many survivors take. Research increasingly shows dangers related to SSRIs and benzodiazepines. This gives me pause when patients ask if I think they should consider such drugs to treat psycho-emotional problems. More often, I lean into the nonpharmaceutical and naturopathic approaches, described below, before considering referral for medication.

For patients already taking medication for anxiety and/ or depression, I do not rush to reduce dosing or discontinue medication. My goal is to have people feeling better, not necessarily to have them off drugs. But if there are unwanted side effects or the medications are not working or not working well enough, or if perhaps a patient wants to become pregnant and does not want to be on medication during pregnancy and lactation, I work with the prescribing physician on a gradual, intentional, deprescribing schedule. Such a dose-lowering strategy typically spans many weeks and months, and I employ evidence-based, natural medicine approaches simultaneously.

Your body might not love a medication, but what it likes less is sudden change. Some drugs, if stopped abruptly, will cause additional withdrawal symptoms that can be quite disturbing. Remember, however, that most side effects are *dose-dependent*. While you may not easily be able to totally stop taking a psychoactive medication, you may do well enough on less, thereby decreasing potential or actual side effects.

I have extensive experience helping ease people off of medications, even those they have been on for years. One key is to choose the timing carefully—as in, not before the holidays or at other especially stressful times, and not when days are growing shorter and darker. Another key is to simultaneously work on at least some of the other head-game approaches shared in this chapter. Engaging with your prescribing physician can also be helpful, though their deprescribing skills may be limited as these methods are not adequately taught.[148]

Before suggesting one of the approaches below, I take time to understand my patient's past experiences with these methods, their interest in bringing back previous habits, and their appetite for trying out new ideas. Practicing *any* of these approaches on a daily basis, even for a few minutes, helps to awaken this skill set. Then, when you need it—say, on a day you're feeling overwhelmed or scheduled for an anxiety-producing follow-up visit or scan—the skill set is there to tap into.

Here is a list of approaches I recommend, teach, or practice with patients to help them improve their head-game skill set: exercise, support groups[149] (in person or online), gratitude practices, prayer, mantras, guided imagery/visualizations, mindfulness meditation, breathing techniques, yoga,[150] Tai Chi, Qigong, hobbies, making music, time with family and friends, intimacy, humor, improvisation, massage, Reiki, and therapeutic touch.

No one can do all these activities, and naturally, many other avenues toward peace and healing exist—surely there is something for everyone. Find something that feels right, that you enjoy, and that will make a difference in your day-to-day life. You can mix and match or do some with a friend or family member. You can also ad-lib and make these approaches your own. If all the possibilities listed above seem unattainable or foreign, or if you feel resistant, just read this section to start your understanding about how this part of healing relates to overall health and immune function. And if you were in my office with me, I'd help you brainstorm about what you might be willing to try.

One key is to practice whatever you choose on a regular basis and integrate it into your daily schedule as part of your self-care routine. Practice helps in two ways. One is preventive. You may notice that with regular practice of, say, mindfulness meditation, the typical stressful events, situations, or challenging thoughts you experience in life have less power over you and less impact. Another benefit is that you can move through the tough feelings faster when they do arise, by leaning into your practiced skills.

Let me share one small example from my own experience. I have historically difficult-to-access veins. I would become very stressed with each blood draw or chemo infusion. I now know it helps to ensure I'm well hydrated prior to any blood draw. It also helps to be well perfused (to have strong blood circulation to the extremities), so I walk briskly around the parking lot or take the stairs instead of the elevator to get my blood flowing. Before entering the clinic, I take a few minutes for deep breathing and repeat a simple line: "My veins are beautiful and open for business." Because I practice deep breathing each day as part of my own head game, it's easy for me to slip into this five-minute routine before my blood draw. I also request a butterfly needle (smaller), and subsequently am less worried or emotionally triggered for my regular blood draws.

Talk therapy and all its subsets are helpful for many people. In study[151] after study,[152] cognitive behavioral therapy shows positive impact on psychological health for both cancer patients and survivors. You may already have a relationship with a therapist, or you may want to find someone trained and experienced in working with cancer survivors. These services are often covered by insurance, and my patients derive benefit from such relationships. Most hospitals and clinics maintain social work departments that can help guide you to providers. Online opportunities for therapy are increasing as well.

Let me tag one skill to encourage you to take up regardless of, or in addition to, any of the others. That is the practice of gratitude, spoken aloud or to yourself—all the people, experiences, and things you are grateful for. Or keep a gratitude journal, or have a regular family gratitude circle. Increasingly, studies[153] point to the fact that being grateful helps with physical and emotional health and overall quality of life.

It's also been shown that gratitude has the ability to strengthen your friendships and relationships, and to improve your quality of sleep and your sense of happiness and life satisfaction. Gratitude also reduces the tendency to be aggressive and seek revenge, while building a deeper capacity for empathy. Gratitude grows self-esteem and allows you to more genuinely celebrate other people's successes. Those with an attitude of gratitude show enhanced resilience, which allows for bouncing back more easily from challenges and hard times, a quality all survivors would do well to work toward.

I wrote earlier about taking up triathlons after my cancer treatment, and gratitude wove its way into my training and races. During my first racing effort, I was in the midst of the 5K run, and my enthusiasm for the whole effort was flagging. I felt both exhausted and a bit bored, so I pulled out my virtual "gratitude Rolodex." I went through my extensive thank-you list of so many loved ones and care providers who supported me through treatment—who sent love and prayers, positive thoughts and cards; brought food; gave massages; and offered expertise with medical, naturopathic, and healing care. Keeping that light of gratitude got me right into the chute and over the finish line, strong and healthy and happy to be alive. Even thinking about that now stirs my sense of gratitude, grounds me, and gives me strength.

As you begin to flex your gratitude muscle, like most anything you decide to pay attention to, it becomes stronger. Gratitude becomes a powerful experience that can shift your perspective, help you become more open to joy and connection to people in your life, and quiet some of your more overwhelming feelings. And remember, it's fine to repeat the same list you are grateful for each day. Often, it's in the very basics of our day-to-day lives—taking time to notice, find, and name these things—where gratitude has enormous power to transform.

I also want to highlight the mental health benefits of work, especially work you find enjoyable, compelling, and rewarding. Maybe you took a break from work during treatment. Maybe you decided you did not love the work you were doing. Perhaps now is the time to try something new that interests you, or to retire if it's the right time and the circumstances fit in your life. Or you may be happy to get back to work and enjoy that feeling of doing something familiar and "normal." Never underestimate the role of work and how it can—especially if it's not overwhelming—be healing.

I remember well my first day back in the clinic after my year of treatment. I didn't feel exactly right yet, and I was still a bit puffy from treatment, with newly growing-in hair. Nonetheless, I felt like a happy kid on their first day of school. I took extra care to dress nicely and pack a favorite lunch. I was thrilled to be back in my doctor chair in the clinic where I have worked with so many beloved patients.

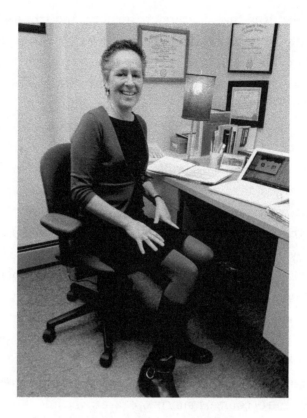

First day back at work, 2015

This is a good place to talk about motivation. Motivation is key throughout cancer diagnoses, treatment, and survivorship years. Those with greater levels of motivation are more compliant with treatment protocols. Motivation is also related to positive outcomes. What drives people to take up conventional treatments as well as integrative approaches, and stay with protocols or recommendations even when they sometimes require Herculean effort? The answer is finding a way to *be and stay* motivated. Motivation impacts quality of life as well as the capacity to evolve, adapt, and problem-solve. Internal sense of self, personality, and history all go into developing a motivated stance, as does external support from providers, institutions, and your family and friends.

It's also true that depression, anxiety, and irritability can interfere with feeling motivated, and few people can stay 100 percent motivated 100 percent of the time. Having drive in your life—from desire for new experiences to being with loved ones, to creative expression, to finding love, to contributing in your work sphere, and so much more—gives people a sense of purpose, which in turn helps drive motivation.

Many of the skills described in this chapter aim at helping find calmness and inviting you toward a more centered presence where perhaps some real thinking and conversations might help define your own unique and invaluable sense of purpose in life. For many of my patients, going through being a cancer patient and becoming a survivor can go two ways. Some people deeply crave returning to exactly the life they had before, everything back to "normal." For others, cancer is a clarion call introducing a time of great reckoning. They now see in clear relief just how far they had drifted from the life they envisioned. They see unambiguously what they really want, and embrace needed changes. And of course, many people are in the middle—wanting things back to normal but perhaps with certain modifications or the desire for some new experiences. For all, there may be the drawing up of a "bucket list."

On a lighter note, let's not forget escapism and activities and habits that just feel good. It doesn't all have to be work, or new, or intentionally bettering oneself. Besides having fatigue from biological causes, you can get exhausted trying to do everything that might possibly help. Let's add to the head-game list: movies/TV shows, podcasts, reading, baking, cooking, a change of scenery, listening to music, socializing, time in nature, snuggling, and intimacy. The list goes on.

The Society for Integrative Oncology has an evidence-based set of guidelines[154] reflecting research on some of the approaches in this chapter, for breast cancer patients in particular. Those guidelines were adopted by the American Society of Clinical Oncology membership. There is more and more understanding that this part of care is essential, which is also reflected in the many cancer clinics and hospitals creating centers or menus of supportive, integrative approaches for their cancer patients. In many communities, there are also freestanding cancer care support centers that address more of the psychosocial and psycho-emotional aspects beyond the actual cancer. Online options are also burgeoning, making all kinds of helpful approaches available wherever you live.

If you remain depressed, anxious, or irritable, where those feelings linger or continue to surface, I recommend specific naturopathic approaches related to diet, nutritional supplements, botanical medicine, and whole-person approaches like homeopathy and/or acupuncture. If you are my patient, I am interested in root causes beyond the cancer diagnosis and treatment: family and environmental history, genetics, other underlying physical body diagnoses, particular life stressors, and how these elements intertwine and play out over the course of your day-to-day life. I am also interested in previous treatment approaches tried, conventional and natural, and their impact, if relevant.

When I work with a patient struggling with anxiety and worry, I look at any neurological imbalances or digestive/microbiome dysfunction. Certain genetic markers can help to individualize recommendations. Single nucleotide polymorphisms (SNPs) are a common kind of genetic variation and may have an impact on B vitamin and other nutrient absorption and metabolism, on hormones, as well as on neurotransmitters related to anxiety. By understanding possible genetic details, a treatment plan can be further tailored.

If your brain chemicals are not in balance, you can feel depressed or anxious. We can test for serotonin, gamma-aminobutyric acid (GABA), and norepinephrine. I then share suggestions on how to get and keep those in a more balanced state.

Another area of interest is your digestive tract and microbiome,[155] which are intrinsically involved with immune function, digestion, and mood as previously described. There is a strong gut-brain connection. Stool analysis and food-sensitivity tests may be added to a careful review of your diet in order to understand more specifically how your digestive process is working for or against you. As articulated in chapter 6, no one particular diet is best for everyone after cancer treatment or everyone with emotional imbalance post-care. Most people, however, will do better with an anti-inflammatory diet and by avoiding food allergens if present. It is often essential to improve the robustness and diversity of the microbiome by including fermented foods in the diet and supplementing with a quality probiotic. Diet has the potential to have a clear, positive impact on mood.

I would also look at your hypothalamic–pituitary–adrenal axis,[156] which is, in essence, your body's 911 system. If you experience excessive stress or are very sensitive to it, you are releasing too much adrenaline over time, and it will exacerbate anxiety and depression.

Other variables can also impact mood. If blood sugar is not consistent, if you do not sleep well, if you overuse caffeine, if you are sensitive to and affected by environmental toxins or allergies, or if you drink too much alcohol, your mood may be influenced. Laboratory testing can help us understand if these issues impact your mood and energy and can inform treatment options.

Certain nutritional and botanical supplements are effective for the treatment of anxiety and depression, including gamma-aminobutyric acid (GABA),[157] L-theanine,[158] lithium orotate,[159] selenium, magnesium, and zinc.[160] St. John's Wort botanical has helped[161] many people with depression. While we use turmeric (*Curcuma longa*) for its anti-inflammatory and anticancer attributes, it has also been studied[162] for the help it offers for symptoms of depression. Saffron (*Crocus sativus*) has positive impact[163] on depressive tendency. Supplementing with B vitamins also helps[164] with depressive symptoms. B vitamins may increase the way prescription antidepressants work, so if you take both, your dosing might need to be adjusted. Speak to your prescribing physician for guidance. Fish oil can be helpful[165] in addressing symptoms of depression as well. Another supplement to consider is hydroxytryptophan (5-HTP), which is necessary to create serotonin from the amino acid L-tryptophan.[166] The right dosing will be important when taking 5-HTP. For those taking an SSRI, 5-HTP will increase serotonin levels, so again, careful dosing is in order.

Research on vitamin D and depression is inconclusive, though anecdotally many of my patients feel much better with regard to mood when they keep their vitamin D levels in the high normal range.

I often turn to botanical medicines with my anxious patients, a gentle and effective way to reduce the impacts of stress and worry. My favorites are ashwagandha (*Withania somnifera*),[167] passionflower (*Passiflora incarnata*),[168] and lavender (*Lavandula*).[169] I might use these in capsule form or as diffused essential oils.

A special consideration related to depression is seasonal affective disorder (SAD), a type of depression most commonly impacting those who live in climates with long, dark winters. Some of my cancer patients report they never had SAD before they were diagnosed, but since treatment, they do. SAD is characterized by having symptoms for at least two consecutive years during the same season and having periods where you are *not* depressed in between.

Like other kinds of depression, symptoms may include feeling down for a large part of the day, nearly every day; feelings of hopelessness and worthlessness; low energy; lost interest in activities once enjoyed; sleep disturbance (too much or not enough); change in food cravings, appetite, or weight; difficulty concentrating; irritability and difficulty getting along with others; withdrawing from social interactions; craving of carbohydrates; and in severe cases, thoughts of death or suicide. It is important to rule out physical illnesses that might cause similar symptoms, such as mononucleosis or thyroid disease.

Causes of SAD are the focus of much research.[170] The reduced level of sunshine in autumn and winter can disrupt your body's internal clock and lead to feelings of depression. In the winter months, with longer stretches of daily darkness, there is a drop in serotonin, a brain chemical or neurotransmitter that affects mood, and increased melatonin levels, which make people sleepier and may also impact mood. Some believe there is an evolutionary cause for SAD: with lower energy output, demand for calories would be reduced during the months when less food was available.

But that does not help us now. For those who suffer with SAD, there are gentle, effective, and safe approaches to keep the mood in a more balanced state throughout the year. Conventional treatment for SAD may include light therapy, psychotherapy, and medications. Add to that regular exercise, time outdoors when there is light, skills from this chapter, and an anti-inflammatory diet. Bring in a few additional botanical and nutritional supplements, described below, and many people can find reliable relief from SAD.

Light therapy is a noninvasive, nonpharmaceutical approach shown[171] to be effective for the treatment of SAD. The recommendation includes sitting in front of a full-spectrum light box first thing in the morning, for a half hour to an hour, from fall until the beginning of spring. It's important to note that light-therapy boxes filter UV light out. UV light found in tanning beds is not indicated or effective for addressing SAD.

Some drugs and herbal supplements may cause the retina

to be more sensitive to light. A person using the drug lithium, the nutritional supplement melatonin, or the botanical medicine St. John's wort should avoid using a light box. While melatonin is often suggested as a useful supplement, skip it if you need to use a light box. Light therapy is also contraindicated for those who have conditions where the skin is oversensitive to light, such as lupus. And light therapy is not appropriate for those with bipolar disorder as it may trigger a manic episode. The herb St. John's Wort (*Hypericum perforatum*) shows positive impact on depression, as stated above, but should not be used with light therapy or if you are taking antiretroviral medication, birth control pills, or antidepressant drugs like the SSRIs Celexa or Prozac.

Research[172] on vitamin D shows clearer results regarding its impact on SAD. So many people are vitamin D deficient, often worse during the months with less sunshine, that it makes sense to have your vitamin D blood levels tested and to supplement with vitamin D when indicated. The rest of the recommendations for depression above may also be considered for the treatment of SAD.

It is essential that your cancer diagnosis is addressed, and that we tend to symptoms that may have arisen during the course of treatment. I also put my patient's heart and spirit front and center, remembering that we are all more than the sum of our parts, that *feelings matter,* and that an upbeat attitude along with some degree of equanimity helps with quality of life and also with health outcomes. Try the least harmful approaches first, and leave pharmaceuticals on the table for when needed.

Patient Story

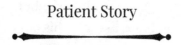

One of my beloved cancer survivor patients, Nina, who had early breast cancer, an excellent response to treatment, and a good prognosis, was nonetheless terrified of her cancer returning. Her fear and worry made it difficult for her to relax, to work effectively, and to enjoy her life. Her oncologist prescribed anti-anxiety medication, but the drugs did not agree with her.

Nina had a history of anxiety, and in her instance, her worst fear had come true. With encouragement and information, she began to appreciate that her constantly stressed-out state was actually not good for her physical health. Nina had been to counselors before and felt she was done trying to figure out why she was so anxious. After all, she had a strong family history of anxiety and was raised by anxious parents.

We put together a plan that included a new counselor who could guide her in cognitive behavioral therapy and develop actionable tools to help. I was adamant about cultivating her daily exercise routine, which was new for Nina. As she got more consistent exercise, she finally understood its essential role for her.

We also added a number of other recommendations, including botanical medicine and homeopathy. With the help of these approaches, Nina flourished. While she still has moments of occasional worry and concern, she now has tools she can use to reduce anxiety. Her newfound capacity for being present in her life, without constant and harrowing anxiety, makes her days more satisfying and enjoyable, and may help her overall health outcomes too.

John, who was treated for prostate cancer, came to me for help with a new symptom—depression. Robust at seventy, John had experienced depression in his life, but not very often and usually alongside sad times like after his father died or with a big disappointment in his work in his forties. John had tolerated his treatments well, with the support of natural medicine approaches, and had what can only be described as a good attitude and a strong desire to live.

Like many men treated for prostate cancer, John was put on hormone suppressive medication after he completed radiation to the prostate bed. From his overall treatment, John lost muscle mass and felt tired, unmotivated, and seriously irritable. He also complained of general soreness and stiffness and being less flexible. I saw that as a metaphor for less flexibility and ease emotionally, too. Unable to do as much as he used to, losing his interest in and capacity for intimacy, and generally feeling aimless and lost, John arrived at my office in pretty rough shape.

At the very least, laying out all the concerns and feeling heard was helpful. We reviewed everything John had been through, from hearing the news of his diagnosis to adjusting to his treatment schedule, to the loss of his previous capacity. We talked about the idea of disappointment and how disappointment was largely related to expectation and how it might just be the time to shift expectations, at least for a while. Because we knew that John's hormone suppression would only be for another year, we set our sights on making the most of this year, albeit with lowered expectations.

I suggested a constitutional homeopathic remedy that matched John's temperament, his tendency for constipation, and his generally cranky demeanor. I also thought he should take a high-potency B vitamin to help with irritability as well as the botanical medicine ashwagandha (*Withania somnifera*) to help support his adrenal glands, as he described the unrelenting stress of these previous few years. We also ordered food-sensitivity testing because I wondered if there was additional inflammation aggravating his other symptoms. As it turned out, he was strongly sensitive to both dairy and wheat, which comprised not a small part of his diet.

He worked to wean himself off of some of his beloved food, to find replacements which, while not perfect, were acceptable. We plotted out a less demanding exercise schedule, and I encouraged

John to accept some of his limitations with the encouragement that he would likely build back up and feel better over time.

True to form, when John came in some three months later, I could tell from his gait and facial expression that he was feeling better. I think it was the combination of the approaches he adopted, as well as simply talking things through and having an attitudinal adjustment, that added to John's improvement in quality of life.

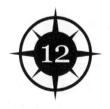

Get Your Rest!

MANY[173] **CANCER SURVIVORS,** as well as those living with cancer, complain about poor or inadequate sleep. Sufficient and restful sleep is important to many aspects of health, and without it, people suffer lower quality of life, depression, and trouble getting through the day. Studies[174] of shift workers show that regular interruption of the sleep cycle can increase the likelihood of cancer occurrence. Sleep helps support immune function, an essential component of many bodily processes, including keeping cancer at bay. Some people have had lifelong issues with insomnia, while for others, the stress of a cancer diagnosis and treatment create this new complication.

If you are my patient, I want to know how well you sleep and how many hours of sleep are typical. I also want to know if you take pharmaceutical sleeping aids to try to find a night's sleep. Many carry side-effect profiles, especially when used in the long term. There are many effective natural medicine approaches. Work with your prescribing physician and an integrative doctor to help you wean off medications, if you can.

If you struggle to fall asleep or stay asleep, you are not alone. Forty percent[175] of American adults get less sleep than the nightly seven-hour minimum recommended by the American

Academy of Sleep Medicine. Beyond its impact on cancer, sleep deprivation can increase the risk of many chronic diseases, affect metabolism and hormone production, and worsen cognitive and motor performance. Insomnia may also contribute to anxiety, depression, and irritability. Sleep deficiency has been linked to risk-taking behavior and suicide.

Sleep helps to maintain a healthy balance of the hormones that control the way you feel hungry or full. Sleep affects how your body reacts to insulin, the hormone that controls your blood sugar level, and sleep deficiency increases the risk of obesity. Sleep deficiency is linked to an increased risk of heart disease, kidney disease, hypertension, diabetes, and stroke.

Your immune system relies on sleep to stay active. Constant sleep deficiency can make it harder for your body to fight off even common infections.

During sleep, your body works to support healthy brain function and emotional well-being. Your brain forms new pathways to help you learn and remember information. Studies show that a good night's sleep improves learning and problem-solving skills. Sleep also helps you pay attention, make decisions, and be creative. People who are sleep deficient take longer to finish tasks, have slower reaction times, and make more mistakes. Studies show that sleep deficiency harms driving ability as much as, or more than, being drunk!

Lifestyle and environmental factors, psychosocial issues, and medical conditions can all influence the ability to fall or stay asleep. I always look for underlying causes of problems my patients have. When they have sleep issues, I am curious about alcohol, caffeine, and nicotine intake, as each may contribute to insomnia. Refined sugar in desserts and sodas and simple carbohydrates like white bread and bakery items also have negative impact on restful sleep. When, what, and how much you eat can also interfere with your sleep. Studies show that even partial sleep deprivation alters the gut microbiome. Lower amounts of microbiota are associated with poorer sleep quality, so foods high in fiber, such as vegetables, legumes, beans, and fruit, which contain prebiotics, can help nourish your microbiome along with fermented and cultured foods. These prebiotic foods give the healthy bacteria in your gut something to digest and help them work better. Taking a probiotic can also help.

The external sleep environment is also central. Noise, light, and room temperature are important factors. Other environmental exposures, such as pollen, dust, and dander, can trigger irritation and inflammation, causing less than ideal sleep conditions. And blue light from phones, televisions, or computer screens can negatively impact your circadian rhythms. Sufficient exposure to full-spectrum, daytime light outdoors is important to maximize melatonin production, one strong factor in helping you sleep well.

Emotional and psychological issues can both cause and be a result of poor sleep. The relationship between sleep and mood is complex because disrupted sleep can lead to emotional changes, clinical depression, or anxiety, as well as other psychiatric conditions, but these conditions can also compound or further disrupt sleep. Research shows that people with insomnia have greater levels of depression and anxiety than those who sleep more normally.

Hormone imbalances in serotonin, cortisol, melatonin, estrogen, and testosterone can all contribute to sleep problems. Additionally, individuals with hypothyroidism, a condition where the thyroid gland does not make enough thyroid hormone to keep the body's metabolism running normally, are also at higher risk of developing insomnia.

Medication can cause side effects and contribute to insomnia, such as those taken for the common cold and nasal allergies, high blood pressure, heart disease, thyroid disease, birth control, asthma, and depression. Side effects are often dose-dependent. Other drugs commonly prescribed for sleep problems, such as Ativan, can affect *quality* of sleep. When possible, and in careful consultation with prescribing physicians, discontinuing or replacing these medications may be considered. It is important to not tamper with or discontinue medications you are taking without careful consideration and support to create, when possible, a slow deprescribing plan. Depending on the ailment being treated, there *may be* natural medicine approaches that can also help enable dose reduction or discontinuation of the medication that disturbs sleep, but please check with your provider.

It's also true that some supplements may interfere with sleep, such as B complex and vitamin D, so if those are part of your health plan, be sure to take them in the morning. Whole-person treatment is individualized and focuses first on lifestyle changes, including optimizing diet, environment, and sleep hygiene; removing stimulants; increasing physical activity earlier in the day; and creating routines. We address any microbiome imbalance with clinical nutrition, removing food allergens, and including probiotics and fermented foods.

If emotional and/or psychological factors are involved, be sure you are working with a good mental health professional to help you identify and address depression, anxiety, and the role of stress. Behavioral medicine, including mindfulness meditation, breathing techniques, or yoga, might also be helpful. See chapter 11 for more help here.

A number of nutritional supplements and botanical medicines are safe and effective for encouraging a good night's sleep. The substance might be geared to lessening stress, to tamping down anxiety, or to lifting the spirits. Many of my patients do not know exactly why they are not sleeping well or even when it began. By using a number of natural medicine approaches, we can generally help improve sleep quality and duration.

If anxiety is a main underlying culprit for insomnia, then the supplement gamma-aminobutyric acid (GABA)[176] may be indicated. It is one of the main inhibitory neurotransmitters that impedes the action of the excitatory neurotransmitter glutamate, which is elevated in those who have anxiety. Taking GABA before bed can help with falling and staying asleep. The supplement L-theanine,[177] when used alongside GABA, enhances the efficacy of GABA for sleep-related concerns.

Melatonin[178] shows positive impact on sleep across populations but especially for some cancer survivors. It is also shown[179] to exhibit a number of anticancer qualities, so most of my cancer-survivor patients take melatonin before bed. One caveat for some patients, depending on dosage: melatonin can lead to very active dreaming—not nightmares, just a lot of dreaming, which can be unwelcome. If that happens with a patient, I recommend lowering the dosage to see if that helps.

Herbal preparations shown effective for sleep include passionflower (*Passiflora incarnata*),[180] a combination of valerian (*Valeriana officinalis*) and hops (*Humulus lupulus*),[181] and the powerful botanical medicine ashwagandha (*Withania somnifera*).[182] Some of my patients also find benefit from diffusing essential oil of lavender (*Lavandula*) in the bedroom. Other patients report help from Epsom salt baths before bed for warming up and relaxing.

We might order lab testing if hormonal imbalances are suspected, and address them with supplements when indicated, including melatonin,[183] glycine,[184] and tryptophan,[185] as indicated.

Insomnia is both the cause of and effect of many serious health conditions. By looking at the whole person, addressing underlying causes, and supporting your self-healing capacity with natural tools and approaches, many sleep problems can be overcome.

Patient Story

Ned, age fifty-two, came to see me because he wanted to get off of the prescription antidepressant trazodone, which he had been taking since his throat cancer diagnosis four years earlier. His surgery and radiation had been challenging, and he'd needed a temporary feeding tube for some months afterwards. "I was an emotional wreck and wasn't sleeping well," he reported. Anxiety and worry about his partner, their family, his work, and finances contributed to his sleep difficulties, as did the excruciating pain of his treatment protocol. Ned's oncologist had prescribed trazodone for him, which knocked him out, though he often woke "in a fog."

Ned was grateful for the help trazodone had offered when he really needed it, but he didn't want to rely on it anymore. He thought it dulled his memory, made his thinking less clear, and killed his creative spark. He also felt that, over time, trazodone was not helping his sleep as much as it used to. He was now in a difficult-to-change pattern of not sleeping, though many of the original triggers that caused insomnia were no longer present.

Deprescribing trazodone should only take place *gradually* to avoid very uncomfortable detox or withdrawal symptoms. If you are considering tapering off a medication like trazodone, I *strongly* encourage you to work with a provider who can help guide the process.

Before Ned began his tapering of medication, I suggested he take a month to integrate a number of natural medicine and lifestyle suggestions to help with both falling and staying asleep. We discussed the need for early-in-the day daily exercise, limiting caffeine after noon, and not bringing his phone and computer into bed with him. I asked Ned to use a lavender (*Lavandula*) diffuser in his bedroom at night and be sure there was fresh air in the room. Since a white noise machine had helped in the past, I suggested he start using it again. I also asked him to take melatonin before bed. After a month of adopting the above recommendations, Ned began his trazodone taper.

When I work with a patient, we taper *very* slowly, over the course of one or two months. In consultation with the prescribing physician, we create an individualized day-by-day reduction schedule. If withdrawal symptoms crop up (agitation, anxiety, or further trouble sleeping), we can temporarily go back up in dosage. It may take a few tries, but many people are able to reduce or quit very addictive sleep medications. With time, support, and a realistic plan, you can find success. It's also best *not* to attempt a medication reduction during known stressful times, such as, for many people, around the holidays, or if the days are becoming shorter, darker, and colder.

It took about two months for Ned to wean off trazodone. He felt very good about it and reported that he was clearer cognitively and felt more like his old self. Not everyone is able to fully discontinue pharmaceuticals for sleep, but many people can take less, which can also reduce known side effects. Once Ned's sleep was on a better track, he wanted to dive into other approaches to help prevent recurrence, so we started bringing in many of the other elements described in this book.

Hands-On Bodywork

ALL HUMANS NEED touch. As a cancer patient or survivor, you are touched plenty, for physical exams, for blood draws, and during preparation for diagnostic imaging. But we need more than that! We need touch that is compassionate, therapeutic, and healing. There is growing research on the positive impact of many kinds of hands-on techniques. For cancer survivors in my practice, I often invite them to consider massage, chiropractic or osteopathic manipulation, and other forms of bodywork to enjoy the physical and psychological benefits of healing touch and hands-on therapies. Cancer centers and cancer-support organizations know this too, and many now offer hands-on approaches from a menu of integrative therapies.

Massage[186] has been shown to help reduce pain in cancer patients and survivors. Many massage therapists and bodywork providers have specialty training to work with cancer patients and survivors. Massage has also been tested and shows efficacy[187] for cancer-related fatigue, a common challenge for many people after treatment. In addition, massage has been shown[188] to help with pain and discomfort that caregivers experience. See chapter 16 for more information about caregivers.

Using self-massage approaches on the whole body can be

wonderful. A centerpiece of Ayurvedic medicine, self-oiling can go a long way to reversing some of the drying impact of conventional medical approaches like chemotherapy and radiation.

While not exactly a hands-on approach, naturopathic doctors have long recommended castor oil packs applied to the skin and used to decrease inflammation and discomfort. When used over the abdomen, castor oil packs can help promote healthy digestion and elimination. For patients that have uncomfortable scar tissue or perhaps a small hematoma from an injury, castor oil packs can help.

You'll need organic castor oil and a piece of clean flannel material, cut to the size you want, in three layers or so. Pour organic castor oil onto the fabric, and allow it to soak in. For a piece eight by eight inches wide, you might use a quarter cup of castor oil. Lay the pack on the area in question. Secure with plastic or use an outdoor tablecloth, with the flannel side absorbing the castor oil and the more plasticized side facing outward. Then lie down and rest. The pack can be left on overnight as well. A heating pad or hot water bottle over the pack can feel wonderful but is not essential. When done with the treatment, place the pack in a plastic bag or container. You can use the same pack for two weeks or so. And then wash, dry, and reuse. The oil does stain, so take care with underlying sheets and clothing.

Physical therapy is often indicated and effective[189] when cancer or cancer treatment leaves behind physical challenges such as lymphedema, cording (development of rope-like tissue under the arm), weakness, or decrease in flexibility and range of motion. See chapter 17 for more help with lymphedema.

Osteopathic manipulation, which focuses on moving physiologic fluids in the body with hands-on techniques, has been studied[190] for its capacity to reduce pain in cancer patients, especially when used alongside physical therapy. Additionally, many people begin or continue care with chiropractors after cancer care and reap the benefits of those visits.

Biofield approaches like reflexology, Reiki, therapeutic touch, healing touch, pulse electromagnetic field therapies, and others often have patients reporting less pain, less anxiety and depression, better sleep, and more energy, according to research.[191] There are no worrisome side effects to these approaches; they are enjoyed by patients and are often available at cancer centers and clinics, so I encourage patients to consider some visits focused on touch, healing energy, and relaxation.

Another physical approach I sometimes employ or suggest to patients is hydrotherapy, defined as the use of water to treat a disease or to maintain health. Water has many properties that make it a healing agent. It can store and transfer heat and cold, and it can be used in many forms, such as hot baths, cold baths, hot or cold applications, ice, and steam. For many people, water has a calming effect. Hydrotherapy can be used to address acute illness like sinusitis by inhaling steam or using a hot foot bath to draw congestion away from the head, or for overall achiness by adding Epsom salt in the hot bath soak.

I recommend various hydrotherapy approaches based on the complaint. Related to cancer or cancer care, I most often recommend hydrotherapy for lymphedema, peripheral neuropathy, insomnia, anxiety, and body aches and soreness. See chapter 17 for more details.

Personally, I enjoyed a number of hands-on approaches during treatment. I would let myself take in the loving touch and find a state of deep relaxation or utilize targeted treatments to address physical symptoms. I continue to enjoy such care now, although I also have times where I just don't want to go to another appointment and months can pass without such experiences. Like many elements of lifestyle medicine, this is an area of personal preference in terms of how you spend your time and resources for self-care.

Many in-hospital cancer clinics and freestanding cancer centers offer free or affordable massage therapy, though it's less commonly offered for those who have completed treatment. With a doctor's recommendation, massage is often covered by insurance. If you're ever feeling a little low, or disconnected to others, or sore and achy, a hands-on approach might be just the experience you need.

Patient Story

Robert came to see me for metastatic lung cancer. He was several years past the time his doctors thought he would make it. He was on and off chemotherapy and other drugs and used me to help troubleshoot side effects or other illnesses or injuries that arose. One symptom that really bothered Robert was back pain at the site of a number of surgical procedures to access his lungs. We tried a number of approaches, but it was a referral to someone who used cranial osteopathy that made all the difference in the world. Robert told me that the first time he lay on the table and the osteopath put her hands on him, he felt a whole knot of pain melt away. He also felt like without the constant, nagging pain, he could move more freely and had more energy.

Robert also used castor oil packs applied to his back for relief and comfort. He would apply the pack and then lie on a long heating pad in the evenings.

Sometimes it takes a few tries to find the right approach for the right person. Like a lot of things in medicine, there is no one way that works for everyone. For hands-on approaches, that's also true.

Reduce Environmental Toxin Exposure
and Support Your Emunctories

THERE ARE TENS of thousands of chemicals, some naturally occurring, some human-made. Chemicals and chemical reactions are part of life. But with the endless introduction of new chemicals and chemical combinations, studies[192] are emerging that should give us pause. The National Toxicology Program for the Department of Health and Human Services' most recent report adds eight new known carcinogens to the growing list, which now numbers two hundred fifty-six. In their first report in 1980, twenty-six chemicals were identified as carcinogenic.[193]

Many chemicals that disrupt normal hormone production and metabolism can be found in our food, water, and air; they are also in the products we wear, surround ourselves with, use in our homes and offices, and put on our bodies. Certain chemicals, such as asbestos, have been shown to have a direct link to causing cancer. But hormone disruptor chemicals are being increasingly studied,[1943] and we've learned that they can copy, enhance, or shift metabolism and, in the long run, may form biological conditions which create greater risk for a number of ailments, including cancer.

In the second part of this chapter, I highlight all the ways we are equipped to rid our bodies of normal wastes as well as toxins from our environment, so if you want to skip all the bad news and focus on proactive steps you can take, skip to "Support Your Emunctories," below.

Public-health and environmental policy[195] must work together, as the environment has enormous impact on health. We need to continue to improve our assessment of chemicals' potential to cause cancer. And we need to make more effort to reduce overall exposure and to better manage risk. Because we cannot control for all exposures, we should employ the *precautionary principle*: if you're not sure something is safe, be cautious and try to avoid it. This is especially true for products in our homes and work spaces.

Here is the growing list[196] of chemicals in the environment that act as hormone disruptors and toxins in our bodies and which we should try to avoid when at all possible. This includes obesogens—the chemicals in our environment that contribute to weight gain and difficulty losing weight, as described in chapter 6.

Here's the list:

✦ **PESTICIDES AND HERBICIDES**, which are used to kill both weeds and pests in lawn, farm, and garden settings, contain many chemicals. Golf courses are notorious for their use of chemicals to create pristine grass. If you play, ask the management about this and express your concern. There are other ways to grow plants and raise animals by using integrated pest-management and organic growing techniques.

✦ **BISPHENOL A (BPA)**, found in many of the hard plastics used across the food industry, from packaging and storage to baby bottles and plastic wrap, as well as in many cash register receipts and some sports equipment, are another source of toxins. Many companies are committed to using non-BPA cans and containers, so try to use these when possible, and when you have a chance, ask stores and suppliers about their practices and express your interest in less chemical contents.

✦ **PHTHALATES**, found in many plastic items to help them stay soft, are a common toxin source. They are also found in personal care products and air fresheners, antibiotics, and other medications used in human and veterinary medicine. Make a special effort to avoid phthalates in children's toys. Concern is growing over the phthalates used in medical tubing, such as the tubes used to deliver chemotherapy into a vein or port. Research to create alternatives is imperative.

✦ **PERFLUOROOCTANOIC ACID (PFOA)** and related chemical compounds are found in Teflon, nonstick cookware, some microwave popcorn bags, and some stain-resistance treatments applied to cloth and carpets, and these compounds contain toxins. Switch to stainless steel, glass, and cast iron, as you are able.

✦ **ORGANOTINS** such as tributyltin are fungicides and heat stabilizers often used in PVC piping that leave a toxic residue. They are also used to protect boats from marine organisms growing on their hulls.

✦ **POLYCHLORINATED BIPHENYLS (PCBS)**, which were banned from being manufactured in the US in 1979, were widely employed in paints, sealants, adhesives, and other building supplies. They remain in the environment in all corners of the earth and continue to find their way into our bodies.

✦ **MANY FLAME RETARDANTS** used in furniture, electronics, drapery, and other home and industrial items are now off the market due to their toxic effect, but they break down slowly and persist for decades.

✦ **CHEMICALS USED IN PROCESSED FOOD,** including artificial sweeteners, preservatives, and added sugar such as high fructose corn syrup, are loaded with unhealthy agents.

✦ **CIGARETTE SMOKE**, both for smokers and those exposed to secondhand smoke, contains numerous toxic chemicals, and so does vaping.

✦ **AIR POLLUTION AND PARTICULATE MATTER** contain a plethora of toxic contaminants, as evidenced by many communities broadcasting air-quality levels on a daily basis; see below for more about air pollution.

Here are some ways to reduce your personal exposure to such chemicals:

✦ **TAKE TIME TO LOOK THROUGH YOUR HOME AND WORK SETTINGS** and remove or replace cleaning agents, personal care products, and foods if they contain toxins or chemicals that may be harmful to your health. Ditch your chemical air purifiers and scented candles. Choose fragrance-free products whenever possible. Studies have shown that many scented items[197] emit volatile organic compounds (VOCs), which can be hazardous to your health. While many of us enjoy diffusing essential oils in our homes, there is some concern that these oils emit VOCs and can add to in-home air pollution.

A plethora of companies now offer less chemically laden products to replace the old brands. And some of the older, larger companies have added lines of products that are free of scents and other troublesome chemicals. See below for more details. You can make this transition slowly; replace items with less toxic ones.

Air pollution and its negative impact on health, including cancer risk, cannot be ignored.[198] When we pay attention to possible sources of harmful air pollution, we can find ways to decrease it in the home and workplace that are free or very low cost, although they may require some effort and priority shifting. Other approaches can be costly indeed.

✦ **HERE ARE SOME TOP IDEAS TO ADDRESS AIR POLLUTION:**

   ◇ Ensure proper ventilation in your home.
   ◇ Be sure gas stoves are ventilated to the outside. If heating with wood or pellets, learn best practices to decrease particulate matter and other toxins from filling your living spaces.
   ◇ Use dehumidifiers and/or air conditioners to decrease moisture, which in turn decreases mold growth, which can be toxic for many people.
   ◇ Review craft and hobby supplies, and choose less-toxic versions and/or be sure to use in areas with adequate air circulation and ventilation.

◇ Be sure you have carbon monoxide detectors installed and functional in your home.
◇ Check your home for radon.

The following do-it-yourself project can help decrease particulate matter. This quick, affordable filtration system is made with a box fan and air filter, both readily available online or at your local hardware or big-box store. Choose a twenty-by-twenty-inch floor fan. Filters are rated by a number of different systems. One reliable system is the minimum efficiency reporting value (MERV) used in the United States and abroad. MERV was created by the American Society of Heating, Refrigerating, and Air Conditioning Engineers, and relates to a filter's ability to grab and capture various sizes and types of particles and pollutants. The higher the MERV rating, the smaller the particles the filter traps and removes. Purchase a MERV 13 filter if possible. Filter performance rating (FPR) is another scale to rate filters. Purchase an FPR 10 if possible.

These filters are manufactured to remove dust, lint, pollen, dander, mold spores, bacteria, microscopic allergens, virus carriers, smoke, and smog particles. In other words, they can remove many of the pollutants that are not good for health. Look at the arrow on the edge of the filter to see which way the filter should be attached. The arrow should point in the direction of the flow of air. With a roll of packing tape, secure the filter on all four sides to the back of the fan, the side through which air will be pulled in and fanned out. Run the fan on low to help filter the air in the room it is placed. Use multiple fans across rooms in your home if need be. Keep the fan on only when someone is home, and mind that children stay away.

Many pollution exposures are difficult to control, so when we can modify our exposures, we should. And remember, most health issues related to poor air quality are to some degree dependent on the type of particulate matter or toxin, its concentration, and the length of exposure, as well as other factors related to a person's underlying health.

✦ **WATER FILTRATION IS ALSO IMPORTANT TO CONSIDER.** Sadly, our public drinking water supply is less than ideal. While it is treated to remove many illness-causing components like pathogenic bacteria and to follow rules delineated in the Safe Drinking Water Act, it may not filter for newer carcinogenic materials, for other harmful chemicals, for insecticides and pesticides, for metabolized drug remnants, or for other items that find their way into the public water supply.[199] Use a point-of-use filtration system at least on your kitchen faucet to filter the water you drink and use in cooking. Some experts also suggest you filter your shower water. There are many water-filtration systems on the market to choose from.

✦ **REDUCE USE OF PLASTICS IN GENERAL, AND NEVER USE IN THE MICROWAVE.** Store leftovers in glass, not plastic. Glass storage containers can be expensive; save glass jars and use those.

✦ **REVIEW THE MEDICATIONS YOU TAKE** and see if any can be reduced or eliminated, as many have toxic components. This is especially true of SSRIs, thiazolidinedione, and diethylstilbestrol, to name a few. Any decrease or discontinuation of medication should be done in communication with the prescribing doctor. When such reduction is possible, consulting with a naturopathic or integrative doctor to address the issue for which the medication was prescribed is key. Note that for some medications, the benefits outweigh the risks, and, clearly, many medications are life-saving.

✦ **PURCHASE FURNITURE** and other household items that are not treated with flame retardants.

✦ **DO NOT DRINK FROM PLASTIC WATER BOTTLES**; switch to glass or stainless steel.

✦ **LOOK FOR PREPARED FOODS THAT DO NOT CONTAIN ADDITIVES AND PRESERVATIVES.**

✦ **DUST AND VACUUM WITH SOME REGULARITY** to cut down on dust and particulate matter that carries chemicals though your home. Remove shoes when you come home to bring in less residue of toxins from your city, sidewalk, or yard.

✦ **STOP SMOKING** or ask those in your household to stop smoking, at the very least in the home. Smoking remains one of the biggest sources of environmental toxins that people put into their bodies. I have cancer patients in my practice who know smoking contributed to their diagnosis, but they still have a hard time quitting. Some feel it doesn't matter because they already have or had cancer. But most research studies point to the positive impact of quitting smoking and removing yourself from secondhand smoke exposure, regardless of your cancer status. There are many approaches to smoking cessation, from talk therapy to nicotine patches to mindfulness meditation. Many local boards of health run free smoking-cessation programs, and there are many online as well. The CDC maintains a helpful website[200] with tools and support to help people quit. It is worth every effort and discipline to stop smoking, regardless of where you are in the cancer continuum.

✦   **CHOOSE MEAT, POULTRY, EGGS, AND DAIRY WITHOUT ANTIBIOTICS AND HORMONES.** Work toward a more plant-based diet, because as we move further up the food chain, chemicals concentrate. Shift toward organic food[201] when available and affordable, as it has a role in improving health outcomes. A review study showed that eating a preponderance of organic food offered "significant positive outcomes . . . in longitudinal studies where increased organic intake was associated with reduced incidence of infertility, birth defects, allergic sensitization, otitis media, pre-eclampsia, metabolic syndrome, high BMI, and non-Hodgkin lymphoma."[202] I believe that the more we study the topic, the more ailments will be added to this list.

Reducing exposure to toxins, if not entirely avoidable, makes good sense. In time, as the scientific data is gathered and appreciated, we will hopefully, as a society, across cultures and geographic locations, create better environmental policy and enforcement and find solutions for habits that, alas, are not conducive to optimal health.

It's also true that our bodies reflect the habitual everyday exposures, not the occasional, so try not to drive yourself and everyone around you crazy by wholesale swapping out everything in your home, office, diet, and medicine cabinet. Start slowly, be methodical, and shift over to fewer chemicals in the coming months and years. Except for extreme examples of toxin overload, the aggregate of toxins over time is of the most concern.

Support Your Emunctories

Like every dyed-in-the-wool naturopathic doctor, I am interested in supporting the body's inherent capacity to eliminate unneeded waste products. This is carried out through the emunctory processes of the body. An emunctory is defined as any organ or part of the body that processes waste and toxic materials so that we can focus on other important activities of digestion, absorption, immune function, thinking, and feeling. Emunctories have an important role to play in attaining and maintaining normal physiology.[203] Elimination happens in many ways—through bowel movements, urination, breathing, and regular sweating. Subpar functioning in any of these areas can cause all manner of inflammation and illness. Optimizing the processing of metabolic waste and outside toxins is something everyone needs, especially those who have or have had cancer.

I wrote earlier in this chapter about environmental toxins and how we should do our best to reduce or avoid them. Ensuring that your emunctories are working well also goes a long way to help detox from both physiologic bodily wastes and the day-to-day exposures to toxins from living in our current environment.

On top of the list of emunctories to support is your capacity for bowel elimination. If you're chronically constipated, here are some general recommendations:

Exercise is central to good elimination, especially aerobic exercise. See chapter 5 for more thoughts and encouragement.

If your stool tends to sit in the rectum but the urge to go is minimal or lost (often related to a poorly functioning nervous system), add Kegel exercises to your exercise routine. Kegels are named after Dr. Arnold Kegel, who in the 1940s worked to help women who had urinary incontinence and other pelvic floor issues. To do a Kegel exercise, you squeeze the muscles in the area. For both women and men, you can think about tightening the area as if you were trying to hold in gas or stop the flow of urine. Squeeze the muscles in that area as best you can and hold for five to ten seconds or so and release. This is one way to try to "wake up" the muscles related to the bowel. No need to do Kegels while on the toilet. But consider sets of eight to ten Kegels, three to four times throughout the day. For some people, additional pelvic floor exercises, or working with a pelvic floor specialist, will be helpful, especially if the area has been compromised from surgery or radiation treatment for cancer or other diagnoses.

Sit on the toilet with the feet raised eight to ten inches on a small box or carton. This puts the rectum in a better position to help facilitate bowel movements. Make a time each day to sit on the toilet with something to read or listen to that you find relaxing. In the rush of everyday life, some of my patients ignore the natural urge to go, and then the urge is lost. Try for the same time every day, perhaps a time you might *tend* to move your bowels.

Commit to a high-fiber diet that includes lots of fresh fruits and vegetables, whole grains, nuts, and seeds. Two tablespoons a day of ground flaxseed works like a charm for some people.

Adequate hydration—think here of half your numerical weight in ounces a day—is essential to support regular evacuation. Use herbal teas or diluted fruit juices to help bump up your fluid intake. Avoid foods we know tend to be constipating, including cheese, bread, pasta, and refined carbohydrates such as pretzels, crackers, and cookies, unless made with high-fiber, whole-grain ingredients.

Botanical medicines and other foods can be used as stool softeners. Ground flaxseed, flaxseed oil, drinkable aloe vera juice, and psyllium husks are some of my tried-and-true recommendations for constipation.

Supplementing your nutrition with magnesium can help with

chronic constipation, alongside probiotics.

For more occasional constipation, consider two prunes in water with the juice of half a lemon. Put in the fridge overnight. In the morning, heat up. Eat the prunes, and drink the liquid.

Effective and regular urination, based on adequate kidney function, is another way we remove bodily waste. You want to drink enough fluids to keep your urine pale yellow. Note that if you take a multivitamin or B complex, your urine will be a brighter yellow from the metabolites of the B vitamins.

Other illnesses impact kidney function, especially diabetes, which may damage microcirculation to the kidney. Working to keep blood sugars in a normal range is important for optimal kidney function. Chronic hypertension puts a strain on the kidneys, too, so using natural medicine approaches (weight loss if indicated, regular exercise, stress management, and an individualized diet and supplement plan) and/or pharmaceuticals is important to address hypertension, which in turn helps protect the kidneys. Your kidneys are central to your amazing blood filtration system and can be delicate!

Smoking affects blood vessels and causes reduced blood flow through your whole body, including to your kidneys. Smoking also puts you at further risk for kidney cancer. Smoking cessation will reduce your risk over time.

Also important is limiting the number and amount of over-the-counter nonsteroidal anti-inflammatory (NSAID) medications taken. Overusing NSAIDs for common problems such as headache, back pain, or arthritis can cause kidney damage, which reduces the positive emunctory efforts of that system. There are effective natural medicine approaches to chronic pain that help reduce reliance on NSAIDs. See chapter 17 for details.

Your lungs work in a beautiful way to take in oxygen and release carbon dioxide and other waste gases that are not needed by your body. Taking time each day for even a few minutes of deep breathing helps clear the mind, relax the body, and support the lungs' natural capacity for detoxification. Diaphragmatic breathing, where you slowly take in a deep breath and fill your lungs as best you can, pushes your diaphragm down, giving your digestive organs a little massage. This kind of intentional and deep breathing also activates elements of your lymphatic system, which helps maintain fluid levels in your body by removing fluids that leak out of your blood vessels. The lymphatic system also plays both general and specific roles in proper immune function.

Many people are very shallow breathers, out of habit or inability to take a deep breath. This would be something to work on by introducing any of a number of techniques that can help you deepen your breath. I wrote more about this in the head game chapter, concerning deep breathing's role in relaxation and focus, but it is also relevant for detox efforts.

If you struggle with asthma, COPD, or other ailments that decrease your ability to breathe deeply and easily, consider working with a licensed naturopathic doctor or integrative-medicine provider for approaches that can work alongside conventional care. Keep up with any respiratory therapy exercises you've been given. Again, smoking negatively impacts lung function and is directly responsible for many, though not all, cases of lung cancer.

If you never sweat, even when you exercise, you might benefit from dry body brushing, which can encourage perspiration. It also feels wonderful, very stimulating, and ultimately relaxing. Use a vegetable fiber brush and move in small circles from the extremities toward the heart. Remember that your skin is your largest organ of elimination, so put it to work on your behalf. You might also consider regular sessions of radiant-heat or far-infrared sauna to help with perspiration. Regular sauna use is associated[204] with many health benefits. Exceptions are pregnant women, for whom sauna use is contraindicated, as well as those with lymphedema.

I would add to this list of emunctories the importance of exploring and processing physical and psychological trauma, or just the sad, bad, angry, and difficult emotions you may have. Tidying up the mind—taking stock and taking time to understand yourself so you can prioritize the things most important to you and let go of others—is part of the process of clearing out internal emotional waste, if you will.

Supporting our inborn capacity to metabolize everyday body waste as well as the outside toxins we are exposed to improves our overall health and creates an internal environment that is less hospitable to cancer.

Community and Connection

SOME PEOPLE ARE born with the urge to be social, connecting easily with peers and strangers alike. They join groups, participate enthusiastically, have an easy smile that draws people to them. Others can be quite happy on their own or with a smaller social circle. Increasingly, medical research[205] points to the positive role that socializing and having a web of community support plays in both the prevention of illness and in quality of life.

This is especially true[206] for cancer survivors. Making this part of the prescription for those who have finished treatment or who are living with cancer is a priority. But how do we encourage being social? How do you get out in the world again after being sick or in treatment? How do you make plans when you're not confident you will have the energy? How do you squeeze in socializing between follow-up appointments and all the other work you do to regain health or manage symptoms? If you're in mid or later life and have not found social settings easy, how can you shift more toward people instead of away?

I think about this often as I see many patients who are not connected much with other people and seem worse off from social isolation. And the cancer care community knows this too.

That's why hospitals, clinics, and nonprofit organizations offer support groups and other activities for patients, survivors, and caregivers, from art classes to rowing to Qigong. Bringing together survivors who, whether they like it or not, share a common bond has proven to enhance quality of life. These groups and activities have been life-savers for many people. Friendships and bonds are often formed, which helps create at least part of a safety net for individuals and families.

Some of my cancer patients and survivors are not interested in connecting with other cancer survivors. They want to go as far away from the topic as possible. And that's fine too. In that case, I spend time exploring what kinds of activities or experiences they enjoy. What did they used to do for pleasure or socializing? I sometimes get online to help them explore local options, such as art classes, senior-center activities, birdwatching, quilting, French cooking, jazz music, or community theater.

Online options for gathering are increasingly available around specific topics, political organizing, and for social interaction. I recommend you commit to two or three sessions to give a new experience a chance. If you don't like it, don't go back. Being open to new or different experiences can be challenging!

Volunteerism gets high marks for its social element. It can also be empowering as it allows you to shift the dynamic a bit, from being someone receiving care and attention to being the person who offers it. Most communities keep a list of volunteer opportunities in the local paper or online. Larger cities have organizations that can match you to a volunteer opportunity based on your interests, experience, capacity, and availability. Studies[207] show that being a volunteer has a positive impact on health. You might want to start with less taxing, low-commitment volunteer activities such as sorting food alongside others at a local Food Bank or helping at a Red Cross blood drive.

Taking classes is another way to be with others. Being in a

learning environment, such as participating in a library book group or a photography course, gives you a shared experience and something to talk about with fellow learners. This is especially helpful for people who find it difficult to start a conversation. Community colleges, community centers, museums, nature centers, religious institutions, and other venues offer lifelong learning classes. Local gyms and YMCAs offer a menu of classes for all interests and skill levels, and we know that exercise has its own separate and important role to play for survivors. Traveling in a group to a place you've always wanted to visit is another way to have organized and intentional time with others.

There are also organizations that cater specifically to cancer survivors, offering classes, travel opportunities, retreats, and other activities. The concept of a bucket list of things you want to do, try, learn, or experience might be heightened after cancer treatment, or for those living with cancer. I like to talk about that with my patients and encourage making plans. Whether a mindfulness meditation or yoga retreat, art or music camp, fishing expedition, or whatever special interest you have, these experiences can help with social connection.

Research[208] reflects that online listservs, chatrooms, and social media pages have offered many people a virtual way of connecting. These options can be a lifeline, especially for those who are less mobile, have concerns about exposure due to a compromised immune system, or spend long days at home alone. Similar benefits are gained when meeting in person as when connecting online. Of course, as for all people, too much time in front of the computer is not ideal, for the eyes, the brain, the body, and the spirit.

I help cancer survivors in my practice explore their community connections and brainstorm possible ways to plump up the social time in ways that feel relevant, authentic, and sustainable. I am also a big advocate for encouraging fun! Going through cancer treatment is a bummer. I often say, "Now that you are done with treatment [or living with cancer], you get a free pass." You can experience something new. You can reinvent yourself. You can try something you always wanted to try. Learning or doing something different, visiting new places, and being with people for fun or on a task all have a way of invigorating your mind and your spirit. You might just make a new friend and, as it turns out, have a positive impact on your health at the same time.

Patient Story

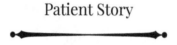

LeAnn had the double whammy of losing her life partner and, not long after, being diagnosed with uterine cancer. She did not have children or extended family nearby and was isolated and lonely. While I worked with her during treatment to help promote healing after surgery and mitigate side effects during her chemotherapy treatments, I was mostly worried about her emotional state and the fact that she was still in a state of grief and shock over the loss of her partner. I knew it would be good for LeAnn to feel more connected, really to anyone or any group.

We explored together her options for an online support group for cancer survivors, and she tentatively joined. She found some kindred spirits in that group that she credits with saving her life. She also decided to join in with a wonderful group of cancer-survivor bike riders in her community and has made some new friends there. When I see LeAnn now for periodic checkups, while she is still sometimes sad, she is determined to move ahead in her life and knows that being with other people is one important step in that process.

Caregivers as Survivors

FORMER FIRST LADY of the United States Rosalind Carter aptly said, "There are only four types of people in the world: those who have been caregivers, who are caregivers, who will be caregivers, and who will need caregivers." I could not agree more!

I view caregivers as survivors, too, who need their own special support and information. While I am a cancer survivor/thriver myself, I've also had the experience of being a caregiver. My sister Joan, of blessed memory, passed away in early 2021 from metastatic breast cancer that had caused a stroke two years prior. COVID-19 had come to shake up the globe, but within my own world, COVID-19 was so intricately intertwined with caregiving for my sister that the lines blurred between the stressors of COVID-19 and the demands of caregiving.

From my own experience and that of scores of patient families, it is clear that *we need an entire overhaul of systems that support people caring for loved ones.* What we have now is difficult to access, incredibly disjointed, and, most especially, insufficient. I am encouraged reading through President Biden's American Rescue Plan[209] with its novel programs and services put in place, including some that support caregivers, and hope it will be expanded and supported by whichever politicians are in place. Hopefully, this pivot to a broader and more compassionate understanding of the challenges of caregiving for a family member will give rise to the sustained and accessible support missing for so many individuals and families.

After my sister had a stroke, I grasped immediately that I was the sibling most equipped to bring her to live in my home. With a background in patient care, I could support her illness management, stroke recovery, and rebuilding of her life. But there was no way I could fully fathom the enormity of the task—the labyrinth of household responsibilities, medical care, scheduling in-home services, accessing resources, and providing every manner of physical, emotional, and material support, all while trying to help a grown, independent person create a life of meaning in a new locale.

You may be caregiver for a partner, parent, child, or friend where those underlying relationships are forever changed. A whole raft of feelings can come up as roles and your person's health and capacities shift. You may be caregiver to a number of people in succession. You may love the role, you may be overworked, you may have lost parts of yourself in the process. For all these reasons, I feel like caregivers are survivors too. Currently, one in five adults in America are caregivers. According to a 2020 AARP survey,[210] more than fifty million Americans provide care for an adult friend or member of their family, with the trend increasing as fast as it can be tracked, as our population ages. This enormous workforce is underrecognized, rarely compensated, and in many ways unsupported.

For families caring for a loved one in cancer treatment or treatment for any disabling or chronic ailment, the sheer amount of work is overwhelming. Hospital or rehab stays are often riddled with complexity and miscommunication. In our family's situation, we were completely indebted to my sister's doctors, nurses, and physical, occupational, and speech therapists, but many were overworked, and coordinating communication was often difficult. Online portals are one solution for communication challenges, but time lags and communication styles vary. Having all providers "on the same page," a promise of the electronic medical record, remains an enormous challenge that often does not come fully together.

And then there is the paperwork! Whether seeking short- or long-term disability status, applying for available local services, scheduling and coordinating assessments and appointments, or filling out forms, paperwork is an enormous burden for caregivers. It's like a puzzle within a maze that requires constant organization, patience, and equanimity, all of which run thin over time.

My sister had three siblings working to support her. We are all educated, we are not poor, and we have a broad and generous community of family and friends who chipped in. I am a physician living in an area with ample health-care and human-services options, with English as my primary language. Even with these advantages, we were overwhelmed and often stymied. I can only imagine how families with fewer resources get by. Under considerable strain, they must buck up and do all the work themselves, with limited or no access to available care, respite services, or financial support.

We did our best, and I know my sister felt loved. We are grateful she found friends, tried and participated in new activities, and enjoyed some independence and self-agency in her last years. But it's a terrible feeling to know we could have done more as caregivers. We learned over time that we had to pace ourselves. We had to take care of ourselves in order to continue to support our sister. I am grateful for the opportunity to have helped someone I love during her time of need. Our sister remained our greatest teacher, approaching each new reality with acceptance and equanimity, admirable and impressive in light of the inevitable outcome.

Here are my main recommendations for caregivers:

✦ **KNOW IT WILL BE DIFFICULT TO SUSTAIN ALONE** for the long term. Seek additional support early.

✦ **KEEP A HANDY LIST OF FRIENDS, FAMILY, AND NEIGHBORS** who might be able to help in a pinch. Include phone numbers and emails.

✦ **ASK FOR WHAT YOU NEED FROM THOSE WHO OFFER HELP.** You might prefer that someone mow your lawn rather than deliver a mystery-meat casserole! Keep track of discrete tasks like this and be ready to let people know what you need if they offer the occasional hand.

✦ **UNDERSTAND YOUR CAPACITY** for hiring, paying, training, and supporting paid helpers.

✦ **CREATE A SYSTEM FOR KEEPING TRACK OF ALL EFFORTS** in the pertinent categories: health-care (doctor's numbers, appointments, test results, etc.) finances, Social Security, personal property, etc.

✦ **ORGANIZE A PLACE TO KEEP LOGIN AND PASSWORD INFORMATION** to phones and computers, as relevant.

✦ **CREATE ONLINE DOCUMENT FILE(S)** that can be shared/edited by others, as relevant.

✦ **RESEARCH AND ACCESS LOCAL SUPPORT OPTIONS** through hospitals, health centers, cancer-support centers, hospice care, online forums, previous employers, religious institutions, and federal, state, and local channels.

✦ **RESEARCH AND ACCESS PROFESSIONAL RESPITE CARE** or coordinate respite care among family and friends.

✦ **SCHEDULE REGULAR TIME OFF** from caregiving responsibilities, if possible, to maintain some of your own activities, to do the food shopping, get exercise, and so on.

✦ **RECALL YOUR OWN HEALTH-CARE NEEDS,** stay current with lab work, scans, physical exams, dentist appointments, etc.

✦ **CONSIDER APPROACHES IN CHAPTER 11 AND CHAPTER 5** to help keep yourself in balance and reduce your stress. There will be times of total overwhelm where having a good cry or a friend or therapist to talk with will be an essential part of taking care of yourself.

✦ **HAVE ALL RELEVANT DOCUMENTS IN ORDER** as early as possible, especially if the person you are caring for is toward the end of life. You want at the very least the following paperwork done, informed by the desires of the person receiving care: advance directives, health-care power of attorney, do not resuscitate (DNR) forms, last will and testament.

+ **BE SURE FINANCES ARE IN ORDER**, too, including appointing a power of attorney for finances/property, as needed.

+ **HAVE THE CONVERSATION WITH YOUR LOVED ONE ABOUT THEIR WISHES** related to burial vs. cremation, as difficult as it may be. Learn what kind of funeral or life celebration they would want, and so on. Most importantly, you want their wishes to be known, followed, and honored.

+ **CONSULT WITH AN ELDER LAWYER/ ACCOUNTANT** who can help with creating the right kind of paperwork and accounts to keep your loved one's resources, if any, safe and to make the post-death probate process as stress-free as possible. Educate yourself about after-death realities related to your loved one's estate. Many headaches and the loss of a lot of resources can be avoided if you have done some homework.

+ **BRING IN THE PALLIATIVE-CARE TEAM** at your clinic. Palliative care offers treatment and support for people living with a life-limiting illness. Palliative care can help with pain control, management of services, and offers some support for caregivers.

+ **WHEN THE TIME COMES, BRING IN HOSPICE CARE.** They can offer tremendous comfort for both the person in need and all those playing a supportive role. Hospice focuses on the quality of life for people and their caregivers in the last phases of incurable illness where comfort is prioritized. We found the home hospice team incredibly helpful during the last weeks of our sister's life.

For many people, myself included, loss and sorrow, grief and sadness, become part of the process even while your loved one is still alive. And once my sister passed, it was also true that those strong feelings were somewhat easier to handle than the enormous, unrelenting stress and worry of caregiving. We will all need help at some point or another, and having been through this with my own family, I am indeed clearer about what I want and do not want, and for that I am grateful.

Patient Story

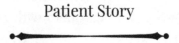

Jo had been taking care of her husband for some years after his diagnosis of stomach cancer. He had a number of surgeries and was in and out of chemo. At sixty-five, she'd spent the better part of the last ten years being the primary bread winner, appointment organizer, driver, support person, and homemaker. They had a good relationship for the most part, but Jo came to see me because she felt like she was losing her sense of self from sheer overwork and from not being able to have any personal time. Like a lot of cancer patients and caregivers alike, a kind of narrowing of life takes place, where the focus is often on health and illness, appointments and treatments. The constant uncertainty of how her husband would feel made it difficult for them to make any plans.

Jo was also experiencing rising blood pressure, which she said was somewhat familial but triggered by stress. She also had consistent issues with poor digestion and elimination. She worried about her own health moving into the future, as she was

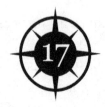

Naturopathic Recommendations for Specific Health Problems after Cancer Care

IN THIS CHAPTER, I share recommendations for specific complaints that cancer survivors commonly experience: brain fog, fatigue, lack of interest and/or satisfaction with sex, lymphedema, peripheral neuropathy, chronic pain, and susceptibility to infections. While I've already touched on most of these topics throughout the book, this chapter is more in depth for each complaint.

Please remember this important caveat: the information is general and does not take into account your unique situation. It is always better to get a personalized treatment plan created under the guidance and expertise of a licensed provider. They can tailor a natural medicine prescription specifically to you, taking into account your physical, emotional, and cognitive symptoms, your past medical history, your genetics, and your current lifestyle habits.

That said, you will find many potential tools in this chapter that have adequate clinical or research evidence and few to no side effects. They will not interfere with ongoing conventional treatments. They may help reduce reliance on certain pharmaceutical agents while helping to create an internal environment less hospitable to further cancer development. And they may lessen or remove symptoms that bother you and/or impact your quality of life.

My inclusion of these recommendations does not mean that *other* approaches are to be avoided. In particular, I have seen chiropractic, osteopathic, and homeopathic medicines, alongside various kinds of energy healing, play important roles in addressing symptoms that cancer survivors/thrivers have.

Many people struggle with late and long-term side effects of cancer care. The risk for developing these issues varies widely and depends on many variables, including a person's age, general level of health prior to diagnosis, other underlying ailments, and type of cancer treatment, including dosage and duration of treatment.

Many side effects are dependent on the type of cancer.

For instance, breast cancer survivors often have lymphedema or cording (rope-like tissue under the arm), heart issues, fatigue, bone problems, neuropathy, cognitive challenges, hormonal and sexual health issues, as well as body-image and mental health concerns.

Colorectal cancer survivors commonly suffer with digestive concerns, bladder dysfunction, sexual dysfunction, issues with the ostomy site, neuropathy, and mental health difficulties.

Head and neck cancer survivors may have musculoskeletal and neuromuscular dysfunction, digestive challenges, lymphedema, sleep apnea, speech changes, dental health issues, as well as mental health woes.

Lung cancer survivors may have poorer pulmonary function, fatigue, neuropathy, and again, mental health burden.

Prostate cancer survivors often struggle with urinary, sexual, and bowel problems, alongside mental health troubles. And men who receive androgen deprivation therapy are more at risk for diabetes, cardiovascular disease, and osteoporosis.

Not everyone develops the same side effects, whether in the

short term or long term. Many side effects impact the quality of life, as well as overall health outcomes, so if we can lessen or reverse these issues, we should try. Regardless of the type of cancer or treatment, the most common complaints I hear from cancer survivors are changes in mood, insomnia, brain fog or cognitive decline, fatigue, lack of interest and/or satisfaction with sex, lymphedema, peripheral neuropathy, musculoskeletal achiness and/or pain, general digestive issues, and skin symptoms.

Whole chapters are devoted to the first two items on this list—mood changes and sleep difficulties—so please see chapters 11 and 12 on the head game and the importance of rest for more. While natural medicine approaches can address the last two items on the list, digestive and skin difficulties, there are so many different ways symptoms can manifest and so many possible approaches that I cannot possibly mention them all here. Instead, I recommend working with a competent natural medicine provider to help improve digestion and elimination, and to help heal and soothe bothered skin.

Brain Fog, Cognitive Decline, and Feeling Less Sharp

Cancer-related cognitive impairment (CRCI) is a challenge for many cancer survivors. On a continuum from brain fog all the way to cognitive decline, I certainly hear about this concern from many of my patients. Often called chemo-brain, it is not only experienced by those who've had chemotherapy. Many other treatments, as well as stress, can contribute to brain fog.

Common challenges include poor concentration, forgetting important details, the inability to multitask, difficulty coming up with the right word, slower processing, and misplacing or losing things. Some patients have said to me they just don't feel sharp like they used to, or they've lost their creativity. It's also important to note that some people were moving in this direction *before* diagnosis and treatment. For others, it's a completely new set of challenges and can be quite disturbing, impacting relationships and friendships, and work and leisure time.

With actual dementia, there is damage to brain cells— specifically, an accumulation of amyloid plaques and neurofibrillary tangles in the brain. This accumulation is influenced by a number of lifestyle, environmental, and genetic factors. Studies[212] suggest that one-third of dementia cases around the world (unrelated to cancer treatment) may be prevented through lifestyle and natural medicine approaches.

Additionally, we can impact cognitive decline by preventing or better addressing some of the most common chronic diseases, such as diabetes, heart disease, hypothyroidism, and depression, as well as chronic stress, all of which put people at more risk. Each of these, on their own and in combination, vary by age and family history and clearly impact, and are impacted by, the aging process. Eating an anti-inflammatory diet and staying active, both physically and cognitively, along with other lifestyle factors are associated with *reducing* the risk and rate of cognitive decline.

There are studies[213] focused on whether having had cancer puts you at more risk for developing dementia. Elements of cancer biology share certain attributes with those of developing dementia. And the impact of treatments on cognitive function continues to be examined.[214] Central nervous system toxicity from chemotherapy, for instance, can decrease cognitive function, memory, and attention, even though the why and how are not yet completely understood. Possibly, the cancer-cell-killing chemotherapy also damages DNA, which impacts brain function.

I've already emphasized the essential nature of exercise for addressing many long-term symptoms cancer survivors complain of; please refer to chapter 5. Furthermore, research[215] has shown that exercise is an effective gene modulator that may positively impact brain function. Also, exercise lowers the risk of further cancer via effects on cancer metabolism. In short, any exercise in the three areas discussed (aerobic, stretching, and resistance training) is the number one prescription to help prevent cognitive decline.[216] It stands to reason that exercise would similarly improve brain fog.

Here are a few suggestions for safety and best outcomes. Be sure you are cleared for exercise, especially if your heart or lungs have been impacted by cancer or cancer treatment. Consider working with an athletic trainer or a physical therapist, especially if you are just getting back into moving your body. Moving correctly and at the right pace will help to prevent injuries. Remember to start slowly and gradually increase the intensity and duration of exercise as you regain strength and endurance. Hopefully, you can also bring along self-compassion if you are feeling discouraged. To get your body back to moving or moving more, bring an openness to trying new experiences.

Being overweight is another risk factor for cognitive decline, so working toward attaining and maintaining a healthy-for-you weight is also important. Exercise along with a variety of other approaches can help. Please see chapter 6 for more information.

Creating and following an anti-inflammatory diet, which additionally helps to maintain proper blood sugar levels, is another way you can help support your brain health. Recall that food allergies or sensitivities can also impact your mind. Therapeutic nutrition through food and supplementation are often part of the plan.

I lean into botanical medicine with my patients who have brain fog. A number of herbal supplements, including curcumin,[217] resveratrol,[218] and *Bacopa monnieri*,[219] have been shown to help reduce inflammation in the brain and to support brain health. Numerous approaches we use have more than one effect, such as the herbs mentioned above. Both curcumin and resveratrol also bring known anticancer effects, as articulated in chapter 8. I love using tools such as these because they work across different systems of the body, often due to their underlying biochemical capacity.

Lifestyle and natural medicine approaches to heart disease, hypertension, and diabetes are all important parts of the puzzle to help reverse brain fog and stem the tide of cognitive decline. It is beyond the scope of this book to delineate natural medicine approaches for these wide-reaching diagnoses, but suffice it to say, lifestyle and natural medicine have shown efficacy in addressing these epidemic complaints and have an important role to play. Please find a licensed naturopathic doctor or integrative doctor who can help you address these common complaints.

Social interaction is another key area for helping slow the progression or reverse brain fog as well as cognitive decline. Please read chapter 15 on social connection for more thoughts on this topic.

Emerging research[220] has identified hearing loss as another modifiable risk factor for dementia. Actively wearing hearing aids to help improve and encourage social interaction has the potential to delay cognitive decline for two reasons. First, the process of hearing stimulates the brain. Second, if you do not hear well, you may be less inclined to talk with others. You are more at risk for hearing loss if you have diabetes or heart disease, or if you smoke. So, if brain fog and mental acuity seem worse after cancer treatment, consider adding an audiology visit to your follow-up care.

If you are a candidate for hearing aids, use them as early as possible; you can adapt more easily when you are younger. Hearing aid technology has improved dramatically in recent years, improving the wearing experience. These advancements allow hearing aids to also be used as personalized, custom audio devices. Addressing any hearing loss with state-of-the-art hearing aids makes good sense.

For those with brain fog or cognitive decline, I underscore the idea that, as with any part of your body, using it generally helps. I will work with patients and families to create, access, and integrate cognitive exercises, everything from reading to doing crossword puzzles, Sudoku, or Wordle, playing backgammon, checkers, or chess, or anything where the mind is engaged. Creative pursuits and learning something new may also reinvigorate the mind and help decrease brain fog and other cognitive setbacks.

Of course, when you do not feel "with it," it can be very hard to try something new. Let go of judgment, and find a patient, encouraging teacher, friend, or family member who wants to help. Or perhaps an online format will work better for you. I've had patients try all sorts of new things, from learning to knit to playing an instrument, to playing online memory games or enjoying jigsaw puzzles. What's important is to find something of interest that gives you pleasure while also providing engagement and challenge and not contributing to feelings of overwhelm or frustration.

I personally picked up the guitar in the years after my cancer treatment. I had played a little in my youth but needed some lessons. After about ten lessons, I went off on my own, just playing well enough to sing with, which gives me tremendous joy. For me, playing the guitar is a good example of my having very little skill but a lot of confidence! It's a great stress reliever, and as I pick up new chord progressions and strums and learn lyrics to songs I knew long ago or new ones I want to learn, I am stretching my mind and learning something new. I am also an avid *New York Times* crossword puzzle addict, playing as many days of the week as I can get through. I relish the longer Sunday puzzle as a weekend treat.

Stress reduction is another key to addressing brain fog and

cognitive decline. Please refer to chapter 11 on the head game for additional ideas. Mindfulness meditation and other forms of unwinding, such as gardening, journaling, and listening to music, have all been associated[221] with enhancing memory and quality of life for those further into a cognitive decline diagnosis; but it stands to reason they will also help for brain fog in cancer survivors.

Minimizing reliance on drugs that increase the risk for brain fog and cognitive decline is another important angle to consider. In chapter 10, I write about the essential nature of some prescribed medications and also about how some drugs may be repurposed for their anticancer capacity. That said, there are some exceedingly common medications that add to the risk of developing cognitive issues. For some of these prescriptions, there are effective natural medicine and lifestyle approaches. When I have a patient on numerous medications and some are for ailments where I know natural medicine works well, I share that information

For instance, proton pump inhibitors,[222] one of the most commonly prescribed medications, used for gastroesophageal reflux (GERD), fall into that category. Similarly, Ambien, an often recommended medication for sleep, is associated[223] with an increased risk of Alzheimer's.

In summary, for those experiencing cognitive issues, whether those issues started before or after cancer diagnosis and treatment, many avenues may help to reverse or slow the process. Often the first step in making progress is to realize there is an issue, and then to bring your concerns to your oncologist, your family physician, or your naturopathic doctor.

Fatigue

———————◆——◆———————

Cancer-related fatigue in cancer patients and survivors has been studied and defined as "a distressing, persistent, subjective sense of physical, emotional, and/or cognitive tiredness or exhaustion related to cancer or cancer treatment that is not proportional to recent activity and interferes with usual functioning."[224] For many patients in my care, fatigue is one of the worst things about the whole cancer experience. Without enough energy, it's difficult to get anything done—to work, to take part in activities once enjoyed, to relate to family and friends, and to do many of the suggestions laid out in this book to ensure best health outcomes!

While the vast majority of cancer patients experience fatigue *during* treatment, about one-third of patients have cancer-related fatigue for months, and for some, it lasts for years. Some of my patients return to their pre-diagnosis energy level at some point after treatments have ended. For others, low energy remains an everyday challenge, and their "new normal" includes insidious, debilitating fatigue, which negatively impacts quality of life.

One feature of cancer-related fatigue is that it is *not commensurate* with energy output and, more frustratingly, *not improved* by rest and sleep. I always ask about energy level and fatigue with cancer survivors in my practice. I think that many providers and patients feel that fatigue is just part of the territory and either don't bring it up or do not believe there are any options for help.

Along with fatigue, patients may have overall weakness, shortness of breath, loss of muscle mass, difficulty with thinking, feelings of depression, and lack of motivation. These are manifestations of fatigue playing throughout the whole system, in my view. Many elements contribute to fatigue, including the cancer itself, treatment side effects, other underlying illnesses, psychological state, nutritional status, and the health of the microbiome.

Certain causes of fatigue are related to other medical conditions, the two most common being anemia and hypothyroidism. Many cancer treatments impact blood counts, and while most people bounce back post-treatment, not everyone does. Addressing any underlying anemia will be key to addressing fatigue. Hypothyroidism, often preexisting or as a result of the stress of diagnosis, treatment, or medications, can cause or aggravate fatigue. Thyroid lab values should be monitored regularly.

Circulating serotonin levels, dysregulation of the hypothalamic–pituitary–adrenal (HPA) axis, and the presence of pro-inflammatory cytokines are among other physiologic changes that may contribute to cancer-related fatigue.[225] We know that stress impacts the complicated system known as the HPA axis, which oversees numerous metabolic, immune, and behavioral elements. If that system is dysregulated, it wreaks havoc on your psychology, defense systems, and overall energy level. Cytokines are the small proteins essential to immune system function and when increased can also add to your level of fatigue.

Cancer and cancer treatment can also impact organ systems such as the heart, kidney, and lungs, which can contribute to lower energy levels. For those with throat and thyroid cancer and possible removal of the thyroid gland and/or radiation to the area, this will be especially relevant.

The main idea for treating fatigue is to address, as possible, any modifiable contributing factors, such as anemia, hypothyroidism, cardiac insufficiency, depression, inadequate nutritional intake or absorption, and more. For fatigue that remains after such corrections, or for which there is no clear cause beyond having had cancer and treatment, we turn to drug and nondrug options as follows.

The conventional medical treatment of cancer-related fatigue usually includes the consideration of corticosteroids, stimulant medications such as those used to treat ADHD, and certain antidepressants. A growing list of other substances is being studied to see if they might be of use.

Nonpharmacologic approaches start with physical exercise, which has been studied[226] for its capacity to help with cancer-related fatigue for those in treatment and for survivors alike. Regular practice of yoga[227] or Qigong,[228] in particular, have been examined and show clear positive results. Please see chapter 5 for more encouragement. You do not need to become an uber-athlete to reap the positive benefits of exercise on your energy level.

An anti-inflammatory diet that ensures adequate protein and healthy fats alongside complex carbohydrates may improve energy level and reduce fatigue.[229] Read more in chapter 6 on how to optimize your diet, which in turn helps reduce fatigue.

Psycho-emotional stress is another known contributor to fatigue. With unrelenting stress, our capacity for adaptation is compromised. We don't bounce back like we should, because we have not had the chance to heal. A cancer diagnosis and subsequent treatment offer their own form of immense stress. This can lead the hypothalamus gland to stimulate the adrenal glands, which in turn generate and release adrenaline and cortisol. These hormones raise heart rate, blood pressure, respiratory rate, and glucose levels and, sadly, also lower immune function, all of which create risk factors for numerous symptoms and illnesses, including fatigue.

Mental health issues can be the cause of fatigue for many patients. Some struggled with these issues before diagnosis, and others experience them as a result of their diagnosis and treatment path. Individual and group therapy can help. Addressing stress, working on removing known stressors, and gaining stress-management skills are important parts of creating a plan to help fight fatigue. See chapter 11 on the head game for more suggestions.

Beyond *causing* physical ailments, unmitigated and unremitting stress and the stress response are contributing or aggravating factors for depression, anxiety, irritability, and insomnia, each of which is its own risk factor for both cognitive issues and fatigue. All elements of our health are intertwined; that's why whole-person, natural medicine approaches can be so pertinent to recovery and healing for cancer survivors/thrivers.

Some people use the term *adrenal burnout*, which is not an accepted concept in the conventional medical world yet, but it sure does sum up how many people feel after cancer care. Research[230] has also found that long-term stress suppresses natural killer (NK) cells, which are important for many reasons, key among them being to prevent new cancers from developing and to thwart the spread of cancer. There are many ways to support adrenal function that, in my experience, seem to help patients with low energy, too. I have written about adrenal burnout elsewhere.[231] If you would like to read up on this emerging diagnosis, see the link in the "References" section.

Individualized nutritional supplementation or botanical medicines may help with adrenal fatigue and overall tiredness. The main ones include ginseng[232] (*Panax ginseng*) for its energy-giving strength; vitamin C for its many roles[233] related to improving energy and reducing overall inflammation; vitamin B complex[234] for its abilities associated with stress and cognition; the herbs ashwagandha[235] (*Withania somnifera*) and rhodiola[236] (*Rhodiola rosea*), each of which addresses mental and physical fatigue; and licorice root[237] (*Glycyrrhiza glabra*), for its ability to support adrenal function and help with fatigue.

Use deglycyrrhizinated licorice products or DGL, which does not raise blood pressure.

Curcumin[238] (*Curcuma longa*), the active ingredient in turmeric, has many positive attributes as a culinary and medicinal herb, from being anti-inflammatory to carrying antioxidant impact, both of which help to improve energy level and overall quality of life. For men on hormone-suppressing medications, ashwagandha and ginseng may be contraindicated. Please work with a knowledgeable provider for a more personalized approach.

In my practice, I refer patients for acupuncture to help address poor energy levels, as it too has been shown[239] to have a positive effect on both energy level and quality of life. I also use constitutional homeopathy, prescribing a homeopathic remedy for the whole person, to help with fatigue. For more information on these two approaches, see chapter 9.

Sleeping well is important; you can read more in chapter 12. There *is* a role for rest, for not "overdoing," and for managing expectations. Short naps may be a godsend for you. Adequate and restful sleep helps just about everything to one extent or another. Many people who struggle with fatigue are the very same people who have difficulty sleeping. Part of this is because getting exercise and keeping a regular schedule are all somewhat difficult to maintain if you are exhausted, yet they help promote good sleep. It's a bit of a conundrum, but you can break into the cycle anywhere and expect to have at least some positive results.

There are numerous ways to address fatigue, and a whole-person, multifaceted approach tends to work best. Sometimes conventional medication will be part of the treatment plan if we do not achieve the results we are seeking with natural medicine approaches. There are many other potential strategies for fatigue, especially when low energy is accompanied by other symptoms and/or underlying conditions. A competent provider can help tailor a whole-person plan for you to help address fatigue.

You may have noticed certain themes throughout this book and especially this section. When we address whole-person tendencies, such as overall inflammation or being sedentary, and understand how such patterns aggravate a host of bodily systems, we can aim both general and specific recommendations in those directions. For example, eating an anti-inflammatory diet will help with mental clarity, sleep issues, joint pain, and fatigue. Being more active will help with digestion, sleep, and pain levels. You can almost predict recommendations when you start to appreciate how everything is connected, and how decisions in one part of your life and lifestyle have powerful impacts across your body, your emotions, and your mind. The more you appreciate that our systems work in harmony, that our physiology is entirely intertwined among numerous systems aiming to work in harmony, and that our lifestyle choices matter, the more consistently you can access a positive spiral of health and feel better in your body and mind.

Lack of Interest and/or Satisfaction with Sex

Physical touch and intimacy are enormous areas of concern for people after cancer treatment. A majority of survivors complain that they have less interest in sex, body-image challenges, genitourinary symptoms that interfere with sex, less satisfaction with sex, and/or "performance" issues.[240] The stress of the diagnosis and treatment often puts pressure on relationships, which in turn impacts the desire for or interest in intimacy. Studies reflect deterioration of sexual health some years after diagnosis, regardless of cancer site or treatments taken.[241]

Many of the most common kinds of cancers, including breast

and prostate, have effective yearslong treatments related to hormone blocking or suppression. These treatments help reduce the chance of cancer growth or recurrence but also impact sex drive and satisfaction. Because the incidence of cancer is steadily rising with younger and younger people being diagnosed, there is increasing demand for awareness about sexual health after cancer treatment. And doctors and researchers are paying more attention, which is a good thing!

Frank conversations about possible outcomes with oncologists, including how your sex life might be impacted, rarely take place during the time of informed consent before treatments begin. Patients seldom raise the issue because most are worrying about staying alive, not about the nature or quality of their sex life. Still, patients deserve to know about common impacts of care, including those related to intimacy.

Having this topic be part of follow-up care, as relevant, would also be a welcome addition to routine visits for cancer survivors. Because many providers are not comfortable with the topic, they don't bring it up. And many patients, too, feel awkward talking about sexual issues. Because so many people are happily joining the ranks of long-term survivors, it is central for providers to learn skills to address distressing treatment-related side effects, and many of the larger cancer centers have created departments where this is the focus.

Of course, this is not an issue of concern for everyone, such as for those who were not sexually active before cancer treatment, who place a low priority on sex and intimacy, or who have had a low sex drive throughout their life. But for the people who are concerned about their sexual health and intimacy, this is an important component that impacts quality of life.

For male-identified people, sexuality is often simplified strictly to aspects of erection and performance, but an understanding of the psycho-emotional state is also important to help guide recommendations. And while prostate and testicular cancer may seem most related to challenges around sex, many male survivors of other forms of cancer share similar concerns, from lack of interest and desire to difficulty with erections or orgasm. There are medications and medical devices that can help with some erection difficulties, and this may be pertinent for some men. But understanding the context of complaints, such as whether a man has sex with women, men, or only himself, can help with treatment plans.

Likewise, for female-identified people, oftentimes issues are simplified to vaginal dryness, pain with intercourse, and body-image concerns, but there are often more wide-sweeping complaints, from emotional to hormonal, to more broadly physical.

When I am working with a patient for whom sex and intimacy are a complaint, we always speak about the nature of the relationship, what the actual issue is, and the importance of communication and troubleshooting, first just with the patient and then, if they are having sex with another person, with that other person or people.

For lesbian, gay, bisexual, transexual, queer, asexual, intersex, or nonbinary people, even fewer resources are available, and this is a skill area where oncologists and allied providers working with cancer patients and survivors must do better.

The American Society for Clinical Oncology (ASCO) and the National Comprehensive Cancer Network (NCCN) have created some tools to help with assessment. They set out guidelines to help providers, including the basic recommendation to address sexual health as part of treatment planning and follow-up visits.

Multidisciplinary treatment via referral to appropriate providers is often helpful. Thorough understanding of the psychological, body-image, and relationship challenges can help guide referrals. Patient education, support, and follow-up can offer everything from basic information about physiology to suggestions for help that show the most benefit.[242] These are cost-effective and do not carry side effects. Both individual and couple education, in person, via telehealth, and through online resources have showed positive outcomes.[243] Hormonal approaches for both men and women, if not contraindicated, may also be important to explore.

If you are taking numerous other medications for underlying ailments or for psychological support, recall that many medications cause disruption in the sexual sphere. Consider a conversation about your medication list with your provider. Are there any drugs that may be less necessary? Or might there be another approach to address the same ailment for which the drug was prescribed that would not interfere with sexual health? Or might your dosage be lowered, where you could still derive benefit from the drug but suffer fewer side effects? Or might there be a natural medicine approach to try instead of the medication you're on? Discuss any change in dosage or medications with your prescribing physician.

Sometimes lack of interest in sex is the same for cancer survivors as it is for the general population—meaning that depression, anxiety, low self-esteem, or relationship conflict, any of which may have been there *before* a cancer diagnosis or *aggravated* by treatment, are important to name and address, when possible, as they may be part of the core issues related to intimacy.

For people who were accustomed to spontaneous sex whenever the mood hit and who no longer have those strong biological or hormonal urges, you may have to instead lean into the idea of anticipation. In other words, make a plan to spend intimate time together, and bring back a bit of romance, or whatever you might call it, to help with getting in the mood, perhaps more from an intellectual or emotional place, rather than strictly physical desire.

Or if sex is framed where the goal is having an orgasm, and that does not happen every time, there may be disappointment and frustration, which can become a disincentive. Appreciating that all kinds of touch and intimacy have a role and de-emphasizing the orgasm goal, at least for some sexual interactions, may be helpful. Disappointment happens when there are expectations, so keeping the lines of communication open—which is not easy for everyone, especially on this topic—is often a key part of helping with the sexual part of things, both in general and, perhaps more importantly, post–cancer care.

Pain is another aspect to consider. If having sex is painful, this will typically be another strong disincentive. For women, pain often has to do with both vaginal dryness and the shrinking of vaginal tissues. You may read about the need for using adequate lubrication during intercourse. This is true. But most women will also benefit from using vaginal moisturizers on a regular basis to help keep the vaginal area less dry. Many available products also contain prebiotics to help support healthier bacteria and pH in the area. The concept is like using moisturizers on any other part of your body. You want to keep the area from drying out, so you regularly moisturize as part of your health routine. I suggest insertable moisturizers, often made from organic coconut oil, vitamin E, and beeswax, placed directly inside the vagina and used at night before bed for best absorption.

For topical moisturizer, I suggest coconut oil to the labial area, perhaps after your shower. This also offers a more long-term relief from general itchiness or irritation and helps maintain a healthy vaginal lining. Vaginal moisturizers are *not hormonal*. Depending on the kind of cancer or treatments prescribed, some women may also consider local estrogen creams to help moisturize the vaginal area (see below). Avoid using anything that can be irritating to the area, such as chemical hygiene products, perfumes, strong soaps, or douches.

During intercourse, use of water-based lubricants or silicone-based lubricants may be essential. Brands that are unscented and do not have parabens or other toxic substances cut down on toxin exposure. Generally speaking, it's better if both partners use lubricant and use a generous amount, meaning you may need to apply more than once if you feel discomfort from dryness. If the product also helps to keep balance with regard to pH, that can be helpful. As the vaginal tissues shrink and are less moist, besides causing issues with sexual capacity, some women find themselves more susceptible to vaginal and urinary tract infection.

Some women are eligible for local estrogen creams or rings to help keep tissue in the genital area as healthy as possible. There is evidence that locally applied estrogens do, to some degree, bring estradiol into the bloodstream. For those with estrogen-positive cancers, this may be contraindicated, although the research is not 100 percent clear, so please consult with your provider. Using oral estrogen replacement or estrogen patches can be an essential piece of treatment, related to everything from prevention of cognitive decline and heart disease to better bone health and improved sexual satisfaction, but is not indicated for everyone. Work with your provider to understand what risks you have, and consider those treatments where the risk–benefit ratio points to the benefit side.

I want to put in a word here about vibrators and other sex toys. More than half of women in the United States use vibrators, and those who do report more satisfaction with sex.[244] In other words, vibrators are not a taboo item, and if you have never tried one, you might want to consider. Vibrators and other sex toys are used for masturbation, as part of foreplay, and/or as part of more penetrative sex. For those with lower libido, difficulty having an orgasm, or conditions that do not allow for vaginal penetration, or if there is erectile dysfunction or motor or sensory deficits, a vibrator may help. This may be especially helpful for post-menopausal women, who may need more and longer stimulation in order to have an orgasm. There are few side effects attributed to sex toy use. Rinse after use.

Likewise, showering after intercourse or sex play is advised for post-menopausal women—not a great action for that relaxed post-sex closeness many couples enjoy, but this can help to prevent vaginal and urinary tract infections.

Sexual health, to some degree, is a reflection of overall health and vitality. As we work to improve general symptoms such as fatigue, depression, body aches, and insomnia, we often see more interest in and enjoyment with sex. Some natural medicines are aimed specifically at sexual dysfunction, but they must be applied carefully, in an individualized manner and under the supervision of a licensed provider, to ensure they do not interfere with any continuing hormonal treatments or positive anticancer treatments completed.

As I often tell patients, if something is bothering you, you should say something. This is true related to intimacy and sex, as well. The more people bring it up, the clearer it becomes that this is an important part of life for many people, and any support, information, or treatment is welcome. I have faith that patient demand for living full lives after cancer treatment, or when living with cancer, includes an enjoyable sex life, if desired. Sharing this concern with your provider helps drive researchers to hypothesize and test a variety of approaches, including those related to natural medicine.

Lymphedema

Lymphedema can be a challenging side effect of cancer and cancer treatment, impacting physical capacity and quality of life. It is characterized by swelling in the tissues, often in an arm or a leg, after a disruption to the body's lymphatic drainage system. Many kinds of cancers and treatments can lead to lymphedema, such as a cancerous tumor or the trauma of surgery, radiation, or infection. Lymphedema symptoms may include fullness and swelling in the area due to the increased volume of fluid; skin changes, including itching; a tendency for infection in the area; a sense of heaviness of the affected limb; changes in strength and range of motion; and varying degrees of discomfort and pain.

You may be familiar with arm lymphedema following breast cancer treatment. Having axillary or sentinel lymph node dissection and/or radiation to the breast or axillary area are all risk factors for developing lymphedema. Additional contributors include having more than eight positive nodes, being overweight, or having larger breasts.

Lower-limb lymphedema can occur after gynecological or prostate cancer treatments. Head and neck cancers can lead to lymphedema in the jaw, neck, and chest areas. Internal lymphedema, such as in the abdomen, is also possible. Other conditions can cause similar symptoms, so accurate and early diagnosis is important. For breast cancer patients, recent research suggests using an arm sleeve *preventively* after surgery can help those most vulnerable avoid lymphedema.[245]

Optimally, you would be assessed for these risk factors *before* treatment so careful monitoring can take place and treatment options, if indicated, are offered right away. Care approaches are similar in all cases of lymphedema, though tailored to the person and their presenting symptoms.

The swollen area contains higher concentrations of protein in the fluid buildup. This high-protein environment creates a welcoming space for bacteria to multiply, resulting in a higher risk for infections such as cellulitis and lymphangitis in the area. It follows that infection can be both a cause and a result of lymphedema. It's important to keep nails short and filed, and to address any breaks in the skin quickly and consistently. Likewise, it is paramount to ensure that the skin does not become too dried out from the stretching and swelling in the area. I recommend using coconut oil or other low-chemical moisturizers. To reduce the risk of infection, it's important to create a robust and diverse internal microbiome. Eat cultured and fermented foods, and consider supplementing with probiotics.

The main treatment for lymphedema is noninvasive, complete decongestive therapy (CDT), which consists of manual lymphatic drainage, compression therapy, and a daily exercise program, along with skin and nail care. Some lymphedema specialists are using Kinesio taping[246] as a way to decrease fluid volume. Surgery is performed for those patients who do not respond well enough to CDT, though CDT approaches continue to be used before and after surgical procedures. Compression (through special compression clothing or binding) limits the build-up of lymphatic fluid and encourages fluid to move to areas where there is better drainage, with the help of local muscles pumping the fluid away. These recommendations show good effect, though not for everyone. In addition, they are time and resource intensive and take a big commitment on the part of the patient.

As natural and integrative-medicine approaches are studied, we find that exercise and yoga[247] show some benefit for lymphedema. General exercise, such as that described in chapter 5, is important as it helps with overall blood *and* lymph flow, but it may need to be modified based on lymphedema symptoms. Resistance training, which was previously thought to worsen lymphedema, has in fact been shown to help build muscle, which in turn helps pump excessive fluid away without creating further risk of developing or worsening lymphedema.[248]

In general, deep diaphragmatic breathing is also helpful for the ways that it stimulates lymphatic flow. I've written about the importance of breathing both in the head game and emunctories chapters (11 and 14, respectively). It can be difficult to start a new habit, like five minutes of deep breathing. Think about tying it to another good habit you have—say, when you are taking supplements, or at the end of your exercise time.

In addition, botanical medicine, optimal nutrition, and nutritional supplements each have a role to play. The herbs astragalus (*Astragalus membranaceus*) and peony (*Paeoniae rubra*), administered orally, have been put to the test in clinical trials[249] and show positive results.

An anti-inflammatory diet will help to reduce overall inflammation in the body and also lymphedema. Monitor salt intake, as excessive sodium may add to swelling.

Ensuring that you are getting enough folate and B vitamins is important, as being deficient will lead to further capillary fragility and more swelling. Bioflavonoids, including quercetin and hesperidin, may prove useful as they help stabilize capillary membranes. Selenium has been shown[250] to reduce the risk of developing lymphedema. Another supplement, pycnogenol, derived from French maritime pine bark, has helped people with chronic venous insufficiency (CVI). While these two diagnoses are different, they share certain features, especially in the lower extremities. It is possible to have a combination of CVI *and* lymphedema, called phlebolymphedema. Taking the supplement pycnogenol may reduce fluid volume and the sensation of heaviness in the legs.[251]

Acupuncture is another approach to consider; research[252] confirms that it helps with swelling and quality of life related to lymphedema. It's important to note that no needles should be placed in the affected side. Similarly, blood draws, finger pricks, and blood pressure measurement should, when possible, be performed on the unaffected or less affected side. Likewise, ensure proper-fitting undergarments and no tight clothing or tight jewelry in the area.

Low-level laser therapy (LLLT) is a newer approach to consider, as early studies[253] show good impact and limited side effects. LLLT is defined as "low intensity light therapy. The effect is photochemical not thermal. The light triggers biochemical changes within cells and can be compared to the process of photosynthesis in plants, where the photons are absorbed by cellular photoreceptors and trigger chemical changes."

Localized hyperthermia, the application of heat to a specific area, has also been examined and shows some results with few side effects. However, it requires special equipment not readily available.

Obesity is a risk factor for developing lymphedema and also leads to worse outcomes.[254] It can be difficult to take up the exercise and dietary parts of a weight loss program when you don't feel well and when you feel impeded by lymphedema. Knowing that weight loss may help lymphedema can be a motivator for some people. Please review chapter 6 for more.

Sauna use is contraindicated[255] for those with lymphedema; in other words, while it may have other beneficial attributes, it can make lymphedema worse.

Aquatherapy, basically a gentle aerobics class in the pool, has shown[256] the capacity to reduce swelling and improve range of motion for some people with lymphedema, even many years after the difficulties began.

In addition, hydrotherapy (also called balneotherapy) may be another approach to consider for lymphedema. Hydrotherapy is the external or internal application of water in any of its forms, such as water, ice, or steam, to promote health or to specifically address a number of diagnoses. Water is used at various temperatures, pressures, applications, durations, and specific sites. Hydrotherapy has been around since ancient times and has many uses across the physical and emotional realms.[257] I have recommended alternating hot and cold hand or foot baths with lymphedema patients to help encourage circulation to and most especially away from the areas in question. Naturopathic doctors have extensive training in hydrotherapy and can help design a tailored hydrotherapy program as part of a plan to treat cancer-related lymphedema.

Osteopathic physicians with additional training in osteopathic cranial manipulative medicine bring hands-on help for patients with lymphedema.[258] Consider a consultation with an osteopath who specializes in manipulative medicine.

Lymphedema left unchecked can cause permanent fibrosis, which is a hardening of the tissue in the area. Natural medicine approaches that aim to keep tissues oxygenated, reduce free-radical formation, and reduce inflammatory cytokines will all likely be helpful, though well-designed and larger human studies are needed to confirm efficacy. These approaches are part of a general prevention-of-recurrence strategy highlighted throughout this book. As you are likely beginning to appreciate as you make your way through this volume, many of the systems in the body that present symptoms can be helped with the application of shared approaches.

Peripheral Neuropathy

A well-known side effect of certain chemotherapeutic agents is neuropathic pain and peripheral neuropathy, which is nerve pain and nerve damage in the extremities. There is growing evidence that certain natural substances, given *during* the time of chemotherapy, can help to prevent or mitigate neuropathy, and I hope these will become the standard of care. The recommended natural substances for prevention of neuropathy differ based on which chemotherapy is taken, as the mechanism of action causing the nerve damage is different with each chemotherapy drug. And, of course, recommendations are only for substances that will not interfere with the efficacy of the chemotherapy. Some people use cold-pack treatments to keep the chemo from getting to the extremities, which has also been shown to decrease neuropathy, but it's not easy to do, and some patients will not tolerate the cold.

Peripheral neuropathy can manifest as numbness, burning, tingling, altered or lowered sensation, pain, and a reduction in strength anywhere in the extremities. This can impact fine motor coordination, gait, the capacity to do daily activities, and quality of life.

For those with lingering neuropathy, numerous approaches can potentially reduce symptoms. The most researched approaches are acupuncture, exercise, topical applications, dietary changes, and nutritional supplements. In addition, stress plays a role in exacerbating peripheral neuropathy.

Acupuncture,[259] which also shows evidence of helping with mood, lymphedema, and sleep, has been examined for its role in addressing neuropathy. Though not every study shows efficacy, many studies do, and acupuncture's low cost and nil-side-effect profile make it worth considering.

Exercise helps with both balance and strength, and may also help with numbness, tingling, and altered temperature sensations. See chapter 5 for more about getting moving. Physical therapy can also be useful; whatever you learn and practice with a physical therapist, be sure to thoroughly understand the exercises so you can continue to do them on your own. Consistent yoga practice also shows promise[260] for helping reduce mild to moderate peripheral neuropathy.

Some of my patients with neuropathy have benefited from topical agents. Menthol in a 1 percent preparation can be applied twice a day to the affected area. Similarly, capsaicin,[261] prescribed by your physician as a patch and sold under the brand name Qutenza (with which I have no affiliation), may be tried. It does have side effects for some people, including rash, itching, nausea, and elevated blood pressure, so please use under careful supervision.

With regard to diet, again an anti-inflammatory focus is best: whole grains, lean meat and poultry, fish, vegetables, fruit, nuts, and healthy oils, such as olive, avocado, and coconut oils. Remember that poultry and fish are high in vitamin B12, essential for healthy nerves. Revisit chapter 6 for further advice about what and when to eat to create the least amount of systemic inflammation, which in turn may help with peripheral neuropathy.

The nutritional supplements that hold the most promise for peripheral neuropathy include acetyl L-carnitine,[262] vitamin E,[263] alpha lipoic acid,[264] vitamin D[265] (for those who test deficient in vitamin D), and omega-3 fatty acids.[266] Glutamine may also show efficacy when put to further clinical trials. In addition, be sure you are getting enough B vitamins by taking a B-complex supplement, because B vitamins are central to healthy nervous system function.

Botanical medicines are studied for their effect on peripheral neuropathy, and many herbs show promise, from curcumin (*Curcumin longa*) to cannabinoid products.[267] Further clinical trials are needed to confirm efficacy, but if you have completed treatment and are not concerned about interfering with chemotherapy, many botanical medicines work to decrease inflammation, promote circulation, and calm the nerves. See chapter 8 for more information.

Attending to the big stressors in your life and your stress response is also shown to be helpful with peripheral neuropathy, as chronic stress exacerbates neuropathic pain.[268] Breathing exercises, mindfulness meditation, positive imagery, and a gratitude practice can all help decrease the intensity and seve of peripheral neuropathy as well as support a better quality life. See chapter 11 on the head game for more details.

For many people, a combination of approaches works best. If you are no longer taking chemotherapy and can bring in more strategies, it often takes trial and error to find the best combination for effective treatment. By advocating for yourself and continuing to engage with your providers and asking for help, you will hopefully find help for this challenging, long-term effect of cancer care.

Chronic Pain

Anyone who has ever experienced chronic pain knows how debilitating it can be. It takes you out of your life, away from your work, family, and friends, and robs you of precious time doing the things you want to do. Sadly, one of the most commonly recommended conventional medical solutions—prescription opioid painkillers—turns out to be worse than the problem. Opioids may stop the pain but at a high price: growing numbers of deaths from opioid overdose and higher rates of addiction and misuse. There is clearly a time and place for opioid medication, such as for certain cancer pain and end-of-life care. But at many other times, we have better ways to address chronic pain. Increasingly, I receive referrals from medical colleagues looking for a fresh perspective or new ideas for their difficult-to-treat, chronic-pain patients.

Naturopathic and integrative doctors look for any root cause of pain and work to address those causes as much as possible. We want to understand your lifestyle, nutrition, work and leisure activities, current and past stressors, and relevant previous injuries—in other words, the underlying or maintaining contributors to your inflammation and pain. We then employ safe, effective alternatives to highly addictive pain medicine for managing chronic pain.

For many cancer survivors, pain is related to the site of the cancer, the surgical procedures performed, and/or the damage the cancer may have left behind. For others, pain is the result of the long arm of radiation. For those living with cancer, advancing disease can cause pain, all dependent on where the cancer is and how it impacts surrounding tissue and organs. But we should separate out here cancer pain from non-cancer pain.

Many cancer survivors are also living with non-cancer-related chronic pain they had long before their cancer diagnosis, perhaps from injuries sustained in accidents or athletics, or from chronic migraines, rheumatoid arthritis, fibromyalgia, or another ailment. The most common conventional medical prescription for complaints like these is nonsteroidal anti-inflammatory drugs (NSAIDs). While NSAIDS can be effective and well tolerated in the short term, long-term use increases the potential for serious side effects, including kidney toxicity, gastrointestinal problems such as internal bleeding, and cardiac complaints, as well as inflammation of the nervous system. And NSAIDs may also be a possible carcinogen.[269]

Natural medicine approaches for the treatment of chronic pain similarly aim to reduce inflammation. One of the best approaches to consider is, not surprisingly, the anti-inflammatory diet,[270] often discussed in this book. For many people, removing food allergies or sensitivities will go a long way to reducing inflammation. Reducing alcohol intake also lowers inflammation.

Dietary supplements have a role to play. In clinical trials, vitamin D, magnesium, iron, fish oil, and probiotics all show promising results.[271] Many of these supplements can help across a variety of symptoms, as described in other parts of this chapter.

The botanical medicines curcumin (*Curcurma longa*), Boswellia[272] (*Boswellia serrata*), feverfew[273] (*Tanacetum parthenium*), and ginger[274] (*Zingiber officinale*) have research showing their pain-reducing capacity. A number of herbs from traditional Chinese medicine also show efficacy[275] for pain reduction, including *Corydalis yanhusuo*, *Ligusticum chuanxiong*, and *Aconitum carmichaelii*, which work to lower both inflammation and pain.

Exercise and physical activity are often negatively impacted by chronic pain. In review studies, however, evidence suggests that staying active is important and likely decreases the severity of pain and improves physical functioning, and in turn, quality of life.[276] Physical and rehabilitative medicines are often important referrals for starting to move again, developing an exercise program, and ensuring you are safe and will not get injured.

Acupuncture has a long history of helping people with chronic pain.[277] It is increasingly available to cancer survivors and covered by many insurance plans. Another whole-person approach is homeopathy, which has been shown to help with chronic back pain.[278]

Prolotherapy, which involves injecting saline, dextrose, or other solutions into tendons, ligaments, or joint spaces, has been examined and shown to be effective[279] for the treatment of chronic musculoskeletal pain. Prolotherapy is typically offered at specialty orthopedic clinics, as well as some naturopathic and integrative doctor offices.

Body–mind approaches are known to reduce the *perception* of pain, which can help with pain tolerance and quality of life. There are positive studies[280] on the use of hypnosis, acupuncture, and music therapy to lower reports of pain. Mindfulness meditation, yoga, Qigong, and massage therapy all show[281] the ability to lower anxiety, which in turn lowers a person's sensation of and relationship to pain.

Communication with other medical providers to encourage understanding across disciplines for coordinated care is very useful. Appropriate referrals for further diagnostic work-up, for treatment support, or for surgical intervention, if indicated, are the norm. I want my patients with pain and chronic pain to know that there are numerous approaches to consider to reduce overall inflammation and pain, as well as reduce sensitivity to pain.

Using natural medicine approaches for symptoms you struggle with, even long after cancer treatment ends, is worth the time and resources to explore. Often, you can find relief, gain back strength, and feel more like yourself. It may take time and might not lead to complete reversal of pain, but the human body has an amazing capacity for healing and resilience when given the right food and gentle natural medicine approaches. You might be surprised by how much better you feel!

Susceptibility to Viral and Other Infections

Cancer survivors can be more susceptible to falling ill from viral and other infections. This happens because cancer can interfere with overall immune function. Also, many of the life-saving cancer treatments take a toll on immune function. During the COVID-19 pandemic, people in treatment for cancer were more susceptible to falling ill. Interestingly, those with a *history* of cancer who were cancer free, often for many years, were also more likely to develop COVID-19 and have worse outcomes.[282]

Are there ways to modify your risk related to falling ill with viral illnesses? Yes! We can modify risks all along the timeline of a viral illness. In other words, there is a predictable evolution of illness, from first exposure to a latency phase, to symptom development, to resolution. And there are numerous tactics that can be used, depending on where we are on the viral timeline. Understanding risk factors, shifting susceptibility, acting swiftly if exposed, and using supportive treatments *during* illness and recovery can all favorably impact the course of infectious disease. This is true whether we are considering the common cold, influenza, or COVID-19.

Remember, our bodies are built to fight infection and can do a good job when given the right nourishment and gentle medicines and time for healing. We are not passive physical beings with no power against even a strongly infectious agent. We have some control in what we do and can take more control with accurate, science-based, actionable information. It is also true that someone can do everything possible and still fall ill or gravely ill, because individual susceptibility is based on genetic inheritance and a slew of previous environmental exposures, choices, and experiences that bring each person to their unique state of health.

We know that not everyone exposed to a virus becomes sick. Likewise, the symptom expression of the illness looks different for different people. Some people get mildly ill for a short time, and others get seriously ill for a long time—and everything in between. Various organ systems may be impacted, to a greater or lesser degree, depending on the individual. Some people with a viral illness might suffer more in the psycho-emotional realm than others with the same illness. Some people fully recover from acute illnesses; some, sadly, are left disabled or, worse, do not make it through. This reflects individual biochemical response to an offending agent. This is why not everyone gets sick with every exposure to every infectious agent. Most importantly, we can focus on evidence-based ways to reduce risk and address symptoms.

For cancer survivors, some of our immune system capacity is altered, but nonetheless we can take up a number of habits and natural medicines to optimize immune function. Many of these recommendations will sound familiar from other parts of this book because, as it turns out, approaches that work to create an environment less hospitable to cancer are also good for preventing and/or treating infection. Of course, there are times when antibiotics, antivirals, monoclonal antibodies, corticosteroids, bronchodilators, and other pharmaceuticals will be indicated, but having additional tools, especially for prevention or treatment of milder ailments, can also be useful.

To reduce risk, we can start by examining predisposition, including preexisting illnesses. For example, we know that people with diabetes are more at risk for acquiring COVID-19 and for having more severe infection.[283] We also know that 91 percent of diabetes in adults is type 2 diabetes, which is both preventable and treatable[284] with diet and lifestyle modification. Addressing the underlying chronic illness of diabetes can reduce your risk of falling ill and getting severely sick with viral infections. And this is true for most underlying chronic illnesses, not only diabetes, so if you are someone who often falls ill with acute viral infections, know that addressing your underlying chronic illnesses matters.

Similarly, studies have confirmed that vitamin D deficiency is associated with higher risks of contracting COVID-19.[285] More than half the world's population is vitamin D deficient. Vitamin D supplementation is inexpensive and carries few side effects. We can impact prevalence of all manner of acute viral illness by ensuring optimal vitamin D status. For cancer survivors, we know that vitamin D plays many roles to help regain and maintain health, and this is another clear one.

We can positively impact our susceptibility to viral illness by maximizing lifestyle approaches to support enhanced immunity[286] and by taking certain nutritional and botanical supplemental medicines. For example, studies[287] show that the mineral zinc may play an important role in preventing and treating viral infection.[288] This occurs by "reducing inflammation, improvement of mucociliary [the little hairs that help us remove mucous] clearance, prevention of ventilator-induced lung injury, and modulation of antiviral and antibacterial immunity." As with many nutritional and botanical medicine approaches, zinc is readily available and inexpensive, and can be used in both capsule and lozenge forms when illness strikes. Zinc raises immune function through your blood but also kills many viruses on contact. The common cold, COVID-19, and other upper respiratory and lower respiratory infections often start out in the nose and the throat, before potentially worsening and spreading to the chest. By "killing" in the throat with a zinc lozenge, you may well prevent such worsening.

Vitamin C and quercetin (a potent anti-inflammatory), which I have written about previously in this book, have been examined[289] and show synergistically "overlapping antiviral and immunomodulatory properties." Vitamin C helps reduce influenza infection by a number of biochemical actions.[290] Food high in vitamin C as well as supplements can help. Again, it is not hard to find these nutritional supplements, and they are not expensive.

Another supplement that can be taken to enhance a resilient immune system is black elderberry (*Sambucus nigra*), in syrup, tincture, or tea form, which can be used as an anti-inflammatory, antiviral, and antioxidant, and has been shown[291] to help prevent flu.

Gargling with Listerine may achieve the same result as zinc of killing unwanted germs. The main ingredients remain eucalyptol, menthol, thymol, and methyl salicylate. In 1879, when the product was created, the name *Listerine* was coined in honor of Dr. Joseph Lister, the father of modern antiseptics.

Mushroom complexes—there are many on the market—help support optimal immune function.[292] Probiotics help create a more robust and diverse microbiome, which plays many roles, including building a resilient immune system. Eating or drinking fermented or cultured foods each day by the forkful, spoonful, or sip is sufficient to help encourage a healthy microbiome.

Garlic (*Allium sativa*) has antimicrobial properties[293] to help support immune function and can help break up mucus. Thyme (*Thyme vulgaris*) is another antimicrobial herb and immune stimulant[294] to consider when treating the flu or a cold; essential oil of thyme can be used in a diffuser or put in a steam inhalation. Lemon balm (*Melissa officinalis*) is another effective herb that reduces inflammatory processes that may be accompanied by fatigue and anxiety during acute respiratory ailments.[295] Take in capsule form or as a tea, or in combination with other botanicals listed here. While it works to support immune function, it also works to calm the nerves.

Melatonin, long understood as a supplement to help with sleep, plays many other roles, such as reducing GERD, being anticancer, and helping support effective immunity.[296] Echinacea (*Echinacea purpurea*) is an anti-inflammatory, immune-modulating herb that activates white blood cells to fight infection and may also be used for prevention.[297]

If you have nausea, consider ginger[298] and chamomile tea, as desired. If you have significant coughing, honey in warm water can help.[299] Herbal teas and tinctures made from ivy leaf, thyme, and marshmallow root[300] have all been examined and found to help reduce cough associated with influenza.

Please know that no one can take all the relevant supplements all the time. First of all, it is cost-prohibitive. Secondly, it's not that much fun. If you need help choosing what's right for you and confirming dosages, or if you want to confirm that a particular product will not interfere with your cancer care, or if you are planning to become pregnant, are pregnant, or are nursing, please consult with a licensed, knowledgeable provider before embarking on any supplement plan.

What's the best homeopathic remedy to take for prevention or treatment of acute upper respiratory illnesses? Homeopathy is individualized to the person. It is the original personalized, precision medicine. What works for one person may not work for another. Studies[301] show that homeopathy, especially in uncomplicated acute upper respiratory infections, can be safe and effective. Remedies need to be chosen based on your individual symptoms. Someone trained in homeopathy would be a good addition to your health-care team.

Beyond supplements and homeopathic remedies, here are some of my go-to recommendations for improving immunity in general, to help prevent or mitigate viral infections. Drastically reduce the amount of refined sugar you consume; it depresses immune function. Eat a healthy diet with a reduced percent of processed foods. Lean into vegetables, fruit, nuts, seeds, fish, poultry, meat, olive oil, whole grains, and legumes. Pull out the vegetable steamer and use it. Grow some sprouts or microgreens. Take time to cut all those vegetables for a stir-fry or salad. Bake something healthy. Learn how to make sushi! Consider elongating your overnight fast to at least thirteen to fourteen hours. This gives all the cells of the body a chance to regroup, to self-correct, and to do the jobs they are supposed to do. It also gives the immune system an opportunity to "tidy up," if you will, and be more effective. And remember, these very same approaches that help prevent or lessen viral ailments also create an internal environment that is less hospitable to cancer.

Stay well hydrated. Mucous membranes that are *not* dried out will flush all manner of bacteria or viruses better than mucous membranes that are dry. If staying hydrated does not come easily to you, consider putting out on the counter X amount of water for the day, and try to drink it. I am basically a thirstless person; I very seldom feel the urge to drink. But I get my water in by making it a conscious habit, by using herbal teas to help with flavor, and by keeping water nearby. Everyone processes fluids differently, so work to keep your urine pale. Aim for half your weight in ounces of water. If you weigh one hundred fifty pounds, aim for seventy-five ounces of water. Measure it a few times, and you'll see what your overall goal is. Don't overdrink—that's not good either! Likewise, use a humidifier in the bedroom,[302] which helps to keep you from drying out. I recommend an ionizing type to cut down on the possibility of mold developing. Regardless, do clean the unit regularly.

Start or keep up with an exercise plan.[303] It raises your threshold for feeling stress, dissipates the stress you have, and helps with overall blood movement so that all the other good choices you make are amplified.

We know that smoking or vaping will make you more likely to fall acutely ill and have worse illness. If you smoke or are exposed to secondhand smoke, it is worthwhile to stop smoking or to reduce exposure.

Bring in stress reduction.[304] If you don't already meditate, think about starting. Even five minutes is worth it. There are endless resources available online. See chapter 11 on the head game for more ideas. Psycho-neuro-immunology, the science where we explore how the mind impacts the nervous system and the nervous system impacts the immune system, underscores the essential nature of this activity. I often encourage my patients to bring in more music, upbeat podcasts, uplifting or compelling books, and positive news outlets. Consider putting a limit on the amount of screen time you have each day, as it is associated with obesity, poor diet, and depression, all of which can make you more susceptible to both acute and chronic illness.

Keep alcohol consumption in check—it negatively impacts the immune system[305] via a number of pathways. This is true for both chronic excessive drinkers as well as those who binge drink. Maybe this is the time you commit to less alcohol consumption.

Ensure adequate sleep. This is a big one and an area where many people really struggle. See chapter 12 for ideas to help you find adequate, restful, and restorative sleep. And you may want to consider napping. Join about a third of adults who enjoy a daily nap. Shorter is better, and you can expect improved memory, energy, and focus. I am an easy napper, can fall asleep just about anywhere, and even fifteen minutes will have me refreshed and ready to get back to my day. Some have suggested[306] napping as a public-health tool to counter the impact of chronic sleep debt! Adequate[307] sleep, in general, is essential for a well-functioning immune system.

If you can, especially if you think you've been exposed, use nasal irrigation or a neti pot, which helps remove nasal secretions along with viruses before they have time to set up shop. But don't use more than a few times a week. You can upset the microbiome balance in the nasal area. From the Ayurvedic tradition, there is a daily routine called *nasya* where special oils and botanicals are used in a nostril-cleansing process, which can help to alleviate dry nasal passageways, among many other attributes.

Try to spend some time outdoors every day. The vitamin D from the sunshine is important, but so too is fresh air, a change of scenery, and time away from screens. More and more research shows time in nature has further positive impact on immune function.

If you know you've been exposed to a viral illness, including COVID-19, consider supporting your body's inherent capacity for healing. Look for chances to rest, to eat well, to continue light exercise, to laugh, and to participate in all activities that help your immune system work best. Integrate some of the nutritional supplements and botanical medicines[308] written about in this chapter.

I encourage my patients to create a natural medicine cabinet, where the basics are kept on hand and can be used for prevention or at the first sign of acute illness. Many of the items listed in this chapter would be part of that collection.

To conclude this chapter, if you are suffering with one or a number of symptoms or ailments since your cancer care ended, consider consulting with a licensed naturopathic doctor or other integrative-oncology provider. You can lean into the natural medicine approaches to find relief and help support your better quality of life.

Primary Prevention, Medical Research, Clinical Trials, Therapies on the Horizon, and Hopes for the Future

CANCER REMAINS THE number two cause of death around the world after heart disease. While there have been improvements in early detection and in treatment, we need more emphasis placed on primary prevention, meaning preventing cancer from developing in the first place.[309] There have been some strides, but we have a long way to go. While this book focuses on survivors, much of the information is also pertinent to the prevention of cancer. Regular exercise, an anti-inflammatory diet, certain nutritional supplements, reducing toxin overload, and addressing chronic stress all have a role to play in primary prevention.

Some of these approaches fall under the purview of public health and should be included in our children's health education classes and encouraged by family doctors. Other approaches, including vaccines and various medications for preventing cancer, are also being explored. See below and chapter 10 for more on this.

I look at an illness like cancer and see it in the context of the world around us. While some people have a genetic predisposition to cancer, it can be further triggered by various internal and/or external factors. Cleaning up our environment, reducing toxin exposures, creating access to more green space and healthy foods in every community—all these are relevant for the prevention of many ailments, including cancer. It can be overwhelming to think about all the work we need to do, but the first step is understanding how everything related to our health is context-dependent; the choices we make each day have both direct and indirect impacts on our health and on the health of those around us.

From a public-health perspective, there are a number of approaches to recommend to entire communities to help prevent cancer. They include not smoking, maintaining a healthy weight, eating a healthy diet, not abusing drugs or alcohol, managing stress, taking regular exercise, and protecting the skin from too much sun. Getting vaccinated for certain illnesses that are associated with specific cancers is another preventive measure.

What I wrote in the above paragraphs took about five minutes. But for a person who struggles in a number of these areas at once, as many people do, it can be overwhelming to even know where to start in order to make sustainable, enduring changes. When I am working with a patient, I try to see which activities and behaviors are most threatening to their health. From there, we start with just one or two suggestions at a time. Success breeds more success. And as you start to feel better, you have more self-agency, energy, and mental clarity, all of which help enormously to start your health moving in the right direction.

When you think about how to be your healthiest, or how to share information with a friend or family member, recall that primary prevention is the goal. For those of us who have already had cancer, we circle back around to that concept and do what we can to prevent further illness, which is called tertiary prevention.

Medical Research, Clinical Trials, and Therapies on the Horizon

Medical research spans numerous fields of study, including biology, chemistry, genetics, physics, and pharmacology, with the general goal of finding or creating new medicines, devices, approaches, or procedures, or using older ones in novel, effective ways. There is research which addresses the basic scientific principles involved in health and illness and can help lead to hypotheses and preclinical studies. There is clinical research which studies how different approaches impact people in good health or those with particular diagnoses. Basic science and clinical research, the study of determinants of health, inquiry around diagnostics, medical equipment and devices, and nonpharmaceutical therapies are all part of medical research.

Some advances made in the world of oncology come from patients taking part in clinical trials. A 2016 paper[310] suggests that clinical trials that enroll more patients help advance treatment options faster and lead to better outcomes than smaller trials. Removing barriers, both logistical and attitudinal, is the goal for those working in the field. While some approaches being offered in clinical trials are for treatment, others are for prevention. Be sure you engage with your oncologist and discuss whether you are a good candidate for any new or current clinical trials being run at your health-care institution. Alternately, in larger, teaching hospitals, there are often doctors or researchers on staff whose job is to oversee clinical trials. You can ask to have an appointment with such a person.

While it's important to be in the moment and do all you can day-to-day to stay healthy, periodically it's also good to get a sense of what else research has revealed since you last checked.

What might you need to know with regard to current treatment or prevention recommendations? Have there been advances that would be relevant to your care?

Translational medicine (TM) is defined as "an interdisciplinary branch of the biomedical field supported by three main pillars: bench side, bedside, and community. The goal of TM is to combine disciplines, resources, expertise, and techniques within these pillars to promote enhancements in prevention, diagnosis, and therapies."[311] Translational medicine is for all manner of human suffering and illness, not only cancer. It's an essential component to speeding up the time between when something is discovered and when a patient can benefit from that discovery.

Personally, I wish advances made from clinical trials and research had been available earlier, as they would have saved a number of my relatives whose lives were shortened due to cancer. The very same diagnosis, if they had received it now, would not lead to the same outcome. Sometimes it feels like we are not moving fast enough, but I remind myself that over time, we *are* making strides; many more people are surviving cancer, and this should be lauded as research leads to improved clinical outcomes.

In essence, much of the content of this book could be filed under translational medicine: I'm trying to expedite the approaches that have research to support their use. When you add reasonable costs and low side-effect profiles to studies that show efficacy, you can safely take up such recommendations alongside current standards of care. And I sincerely hope these kinds of guidelines will be integrated into the National Comprehensive Cancer Network (NCCN) Guidelines discussed below.

Therapies on the Horizon

The future of cancer care is shifting rapidly, and in the coming decades everything from targeted vaccines to personalized immunotherapy, to more focus on the role of the microbiome, will become the standard of care. Meanwhile, for survivors there are a number of approaches that are less available, have less research to support their efficacy, and are less known. I place this section here for completion's sake and with the understanding that over time, it is likely that these and additional interventions will prove important for cancer survivors as well as clinicians to know about and consider. The topics I will address are hyperthermia and IV nutrition.

Hyperthermia

We know that fever is the body's natural response to pathogens and other disease processes. For over 5,000 years people have intentionally used fever to help the body fight infection and other ailments. It is a highly evolved and complicated process we learn more about the more it's studied. In 1891, working at Sloan Kettering, William Coley published a paper touting the potential positive impact of therapeutic fever. I learned in naturopathic school about Coley's toxins,[312] but not much more.

There are numerous examples through history of patients getting better from a more serious condition after having a high fever. There is also a body of research showing that those with fewer incidences of fever over a lifetime have a higher incidence of cancer. We know that physiologically, fever is an essential part of fighting all kinds of disease, by improving immune response to infection. Yet because fevers make people uncomfortable, parents reach for fever-lowering medication for children, and adults regularly do away with fevers by taking acetaminophen or ibuprofen. It is safe to say we would probably do better overall if we allowed our bodies, as appropriate, to experience the occasional fever.

Of course, very high fevers can put you or a child at risk for a febrile seizure, delirium, or actual tissue damage, and these fevers must be managed. Most fevers, however, do not reach that high. We need to rebrand fevers as a tool the body uses to fight infection, as opposed to the enemy that needs to be suppressed. Fever, like any symptom, must always be appreciated in the overall context of the person's health at a moment in time. For cancer survivors, having the once-in-a-while fever, or seeking out options for hyperthermia, may well be an excellent way to support innate immune function.

There are two main forms of hyperthermia: local/regional hyperthermia and full-body fever therapy. With locoregional hyperthermia (LRHT), a specific kind of heat is applied to a region of the body, usually the area where a tumor was located or a recurrence has taken place. The LRHT therapy is used in some United States hospitals to help enhance efficacy of treatment.[313] During cancer care, hyperthermia is aimed at killing malignant cells and also can help to enhance other conventional therapies and complementary therapies, including chemotherapy, radiotherapy, immunotherapy, targeted therapies, IV ascorbic acid, and others.

Typically, the patient lies supine on a slim water mattress. Conductive metal panels are above and below, covered with water bladders placed directly on the skin. The machine slowly heats the tissues between the probes to between 40 and 43°C (or 104 to 109.5°F). Often done simultaneously with IV vitamin C, alpha lipoic acid, or other chemical or natural agents to which the patient has shown sensitivity, most sessions last about an hour.

What is taking place? The heat drives circulation to the area, which for those in treatment may enhance chemotherapy as well as targeted naturopathic anticancer agents. The warmth also drives circulation *away* from places it is not needed, thereby decreasing potential toxicity at the same time. For those who have completed treatment, LRHT can slow tumor angiogenesis, due to enhanced oxygenation to the areas in question. Blood vessels that carry nutrients to cancer cells do not like heat, so their function is compromised. Cancer cells produce heat-shock proteins, which stick to the surface of cancer cells and act as a sign for the immune system to recognize the cancer cells, which causes an immune-stimulating response.[314]

Full-body hyperthermia, sometimes called body-warming treatment, has been shown to be safe and well tolerated. Studied alongside chemotherapy (thermochemotherapy), it may enhance efficacy of treatment and protect the rest of the body. Efficacy in this realm comes from fever's ability to increase perfusion, thereby getting chemotherapy more reliably where it needs to go.

How is this treatment administered? Using external heating devices (as opposed to other disease processes that raise fever), the goal is to attain fever range (38.5 to 40.5°C, or 101.3 to 104.9°F) and to stay there for several hours, depending on treatment protocols. For survivors, these approaches are used with an eye toward preventing recurrence. Intermittent treatment is a way to stimulate immune function and potentially clear cancer cells that might be trying to establish a new cancer site.

There are contraindications for full-body hyperthermia, such as arrythmia, thrombocytopenia (not enough platelets), severe anemia, bleeding disorders, active brain lesions, severe pleural effusion or edema, and possibly liver or kidney disease.

The prep for full-body hyperthermia includes at least a six-hour fast, Fleet Enema, extra hydration, full-body coverage with loose-fitting, pajama-like tops and bottoms to avoid burning, as well as emptying the bladder. An IV is inserted for the fluids saline and dextrose to prevent dehydration and hypoglycemia. A rectal thermometer is inserted and EKG leads are placed. The patient is monitored throughout treatment for pulse and respiration, oximetry, heart rate, and blood pressure, as well as an EKG.

Administration of treatment varies based on provider and machine protocols. It might take two to three hours to raise the core temperature to between 38.5 and 40.5°C. The patient would maintain that temperature for one to two hours, followed by a cooling phase for another one to two hours. Most people feel quite well afterward—warm and tired, but otherwise fine.

There is an additional way the fever state can be attained for the purpose of fighting cancer, which is by intentional exposure to fever-causing substances. Interleukin-2 has been studied[315] for this method and shows promise in the treatment of malignant melanoma. This method carries the potential for dangerous side effects and needs to be closely managed. Further research and clinical trials are needed before such techniques are widely recommended or adopted in the treatment of cancer patients, or for survivors looking for more proactive, preventive medicine.

I have personally taken advantage of each method of hyperthermia in the years since my own treatment. I will take a week where I do four days of LRHT and then a middle day of full-body hyperthermia. I cannot say I look forward to these days, and it does cost time and money. That said, using these additional approaches to stimulate my immune function, and to lean into another innate healing capacity in my body, feels worth the time and effort.

We need more clinical trials that use hyperthermia in order to test efficacy both for current cancer patients and for survivors with an eye to preventing recurrence. We need more clinics and clinicians trained in these approaches and who have access to state-of-the-art hyperthermia technology. This area is ripe with opportunities for research on basic science components and in clinics with patients who are looking to further engage their inborn mechanisms for healing. I also believe there is tremendous potential for collaborative work and enhancing efficacy of both conventional and naturopathic oncology treatments by using hyperthermia.

IV Nutrients

Interest in the use of IV nutritional supplements in the treatment of cancer is growing. We can extrapolate that it might also be indicated for those wanting to prevent recurrence. Vitamin C in particular has been studied and shows some promising results.[316] Similar to many natural or integrative approaches to cancer or to prevention of recurrence, we need more well-designed, controlled studies to help us further determine who will most benefit from IV supplementation. Adoption of such approaches will follow the research, so hopefully in the coming years there will be more and better research to help inform clinical options.

Some people do not like needles and do not feel well with IVs related to fluid balance in the body, but most people tolerate these treatments well. For those who have a port in place, IV nutrients can also be delivered through a port. I have had IVs over the course of my treatment and afterward. Like many approaches, time and resources are involved, and most insurance companies will not reimburse for IV therapies. Many naturopathic doctors who specialize in oncology will offer IV therapies as part of a treatment approach.

Beyond hyperthermia and the use of IV nutrition, other substances and techniques will be discovered and evolve over time. Research into novel approaches takes curiosity and willingness to look broadly at the world around us, to develop hypotheses and test them as we continue to look for ways to help people address symptoms and prevent recurrence. There are so many areas in health and medicine deserving of our research intelligence and dollars, and hopefully actionable information related to best-health survivorship will be high on the list.

Hopes for the Future

Since the early 2000s there has been a growing interest in integrative oncology, further powered by patient interest and desire. The scientific evidence is also catching up with many recommendations that naturopathic doctors and other integrative providers have been sharing for decades.

When I first started writing about my experiences right after diagnosis and during treatment, it became part of my healing to let people know how much more they could do during treatment to support conventional care and prevent or, when needed, address side effects that arose. I saw both as a patient sharing from my experience and from the many patients in my care how much it helped to have a conversation, to learn about relevant research, to have support and love and guidance, especially when I hit a bump in the road, which happens for most every cancer patient from time to time. I feel tremendously lucky to have had the naturopathic and integrative medicine team, which I sought, in addition to and separate from my top-notch oncology team at Massachusetts General Hospital in Boston.

There are not enough naturopathic doctors or those

trained in integrative oncology for every person in treatment or afterward. This book is part of a bridge to that time. Most large cancer centers appreciate the research that reflects how integrative medicine strategies help with both quality of life and health outcomes. Integrative approaches such as yoga, massage, meditation, and other offerings are more and more common for cancer patients and survivors. Most cancer centers also have nutritionists on hand. Physical therapy prescriptions can be made when indicated for musculoskeletal symptoms related to cancer or cancer care. Mental health counselors and social workers are also part of many cancer care facilities. These are all excellent and essential steps in the right direction, and, hopefully, you or your loved ones have accessed these various kinds of support as needed. You don't have to go through this alone. And as studies reveal, these kinds of approaches, beyond just being supportive, impact both quality of life and health outcomes.

We also need to champion some of the other approaches described in this book so that every cancer patient knows steps they can take to help create an internal environment least hospitable to cancer. I want every survivor to know there are approaches to try when side effects from treatment last well beyond the end of care. I want my patients' health-care teams to be out front with the research, and to share and encourage lifestyle medicine alongside other effective and promising methods. My vision is that once you work with your oncologist, you go next door and work with your naturopathic doctor or a medical doctor with advanced training in integrative oncology. I see this as a necessary norm.

There are some examples of this already, but we need more, we need funding, we need education, and we need research. We need to test botanical medicines and specific diets or nutritional supplements side by side with conventional drugs—not to replace the current standards of care but to reap the most benefit from a more integrated approach. And we need multicenter studies with large numbers of participants to develop evidence-based best practices. We need to destigmatize cancer in general *and* the use of natural medicines to help during and after care.

I believe this is forthcoming, mostly because of an educated and demanding public. The age of the passive patient is further and further behind us. People do their own research and want their doctors on board. The trend for cancer patients using at least one form of natural medicine during and after their care continues to rise. Let's get this work coordinated and lean into those approaches that are individualized to the patient, the kind of cancer they had, the impacts of their treatment, and their temperament. Let's create a medical model[317] where it's not either-or but "yes, and"!

If you've been through cancer care, your oncologists likely followed the National Comprehensive Cancer Network (NCCN) Guidelines. This resource is the gold standard that guides conventional care and is used by oncology teams around the globe. Recommendations include those related to prevention, diagnosis, treatment, and management of cancer at every stage of disease. NCCN Guidelines are continuously reviewed and updated based on a critical review by cancer experts following NCCN criteria of evidence and consensus. Recommendations are made only upon the method achieving the highest categories of evidence. That said, they include approaches that are *in the pipeline for consideration*—in other words, approaches that would fall under potential future recommendations. I hope that much of the content of this book, and all the many studies referenced, will help inform consideration for inclusion in NCCN Guidelines, even if not yet at the highest level of evidence.

This would at least create an opportunity for the world of oncology researchers to become aware of these approaches and their benefit for patients. This could help the development of large-scale clinical trials, one essential component to being included as a recommendation in the NCCN Guidelines. Interest in and funding for such studies is long overdue.

I am an optimistic person, and research[318] reflects that the general population of doctors is open to recommending natural medicine approaches more than at any other time in history. Doctors are likely to be more open to patients pursuing natural medicine care alongside their conventional care. Interestingly, as more physicians age and receive a cancer diagnosis, they too are more open to how else they can support their health alongside conventional treatment. Medical doctors who are patients in my naturopathic practice have gone from deeply skeptical to curious to enthusiastic over the course of their cancer treatment. I am glad to be part of a growing cadre of providers who continue to open this door and bring in all who are interested, for the ultimate benefit of our patients.

As for you, if you have finished cancer treatment, I hope you mark the moment. Sometimes the pomp and circumstance of a formal graduation from a long effort can seem affected or pretentious. But finishing up cancer treatment is another example of how we are all graduating from one thing or another at any given moment in life: a recent challenge, a course of study, a phase of life evolving to the next, a job or relationship shift, an accomplishment big or small, or simply a realization that shifts our focus or changes the course of our own river of life.

It is my deepest hope that this book be a helpful resource as you navigate forward on your healing path. May we each find the right information at the right time, a well of inspiration when we need it, and the essential comfort and support of loved ones, so essential to our healing. Here's to your vibrant health!

Acknowledgments

I HAVE HAD the great fortune to have many people who believe in me and help chart my course through life. Family, friends, colleagues, and my health care team all helped inspire and guide the evolution and creation of this book.

For the man at my side, Paul Herscu, ND, MPH, indefatigable, dedicated, loving, and strong, I would not be here today without you. Literally. For your care and compassion through good times and tough times, for your suggestions on this manuscript, for your unwavering support, I am forever grateful. Thank you for giving me all the time and space I need to be me and for joining me on our amazing life adventure. To our grown children, Sophia, Misha, and Jonah Herscu, for your unconditional love, for your good humor and support, and most especially for helping define my purpose-driven life.

To the devoted women who help support my work: Kimberly McGuire, Linda Smith, and Diana Venman, who oversee many of the details, large and small, of my work life, which allows me to focus on my patients, teaching, writing, my family, and other community-building and creative pursuits.

To Tina Kaczor, ND, FABNO, who offered encouragement early and throughout for this project and lent her considerable knowledge to many of my questions. To Mitzi Lebensorger, who has edited much of my writing since the 1980s, with a fine eye and generous spirit, and who reviewed this manuscript and offered a mother lode of helpful suggestions and clarifications. To Bonnie Diamond, MAc, for sharing her acupuncture patient story.

To my people Lynn Curry, Lynn Bowmaster and Michael Docter, Deb Habib and Ricky Baruch, Leslie Cooperband and Wes Jarrell, John Clayton and Sharon Clayton-Dunn, Julieanne Forbes, ND, and Ange DiBennedetto, for enduring love and friendship; to my book-group buddies: Lee MacKinnon, Susan Loring-Wells, Wendy Kohler, Alessandra Mucci-Ramos, Jaymie Chernoff, Sue Morrello, Stacey Lennard, and Deb Habib (again!) for your kindnesses and camaraderie. To the crew at the Institute for Natural Medicine during my years there: Michelle Simon, PhD, ND; Kim Stewart; Griffin McMath, ND; Leigh Delano; and Kelsang Tenpa—who taught me the pleasure of working on a team with a sense of shared vision.

To my care providers, thank you for your intelligence, compassion, and expertise and for putting up with my endless questions, discussions, and ideas: Jacob Schor, ND, FABNO; Tina Kaczor, ND, FABNO; Gurdev Parmar, ND, FABNO; Kyle Cronin, ND, Michael Cronin, ND; the late Ralf Kleefe, MD; Lindsay Rockwell, DO; Orion Howard, MD; A. K. Goodman, MD; Richard Penson, MD; Barbara Smith, MD, PhD; Beverly Moy, MD, PhD; Amy Colwell, MD; Raul Uppot, MD; Alphonse Taghian, MD, PhD; and to Linda Levine, DC, for your magical healing hands and openhearted nature.

To the early readers of this manuscript, including each generous person who offered constructive criticism and praise—thank you for your time, expertise, feedback, and good cheer. Special thanks to Renee Rossi, MD, MFA, MA-Ay, for suggestions related to Ayurvedic medicine, and Paul Mittman, ND, EDD, and

Linda Bornstien, MD, another of my wonderful providers, who also offered content feedback on early renditions of this manuscript.

To my agent, Nancy Rosenfeld, at AAA Books Unlimited for her early enthusiasm, attention to detail, and her dogged determination. To John Koehler at Koehler Books for believing in this project and overseeing its completion. To my book editor, Hannah Woodlan, for her fine eye and clarifying suggestions. To Danielle Koehler for creating my author website and for the beautiful design of the book.

To my patients who have been through cancer, and really, to all my patients, thank you for allowing me the privilege to be your doctor, to learn about your life, your sorrow, your pain, your joy, and for illuminating the resilience of the human spirit. I love my work with you and hope I have helped you evolve as much as you have helped me. And to the people I do not know who read my writing or hear me speak and send feedback and appreciation, you keep me learning and in the writer's chair. Thank you!

And to my siblings, whom I've shared a life with, David Rothenberg and Lauren Comando, Nancy Rothenberg and Eric Conz, and the late Joan Rothenberg, and most especially to my parents, Doris Cynthia Jaffe Rothenberg and Harry Rothenberg, who never got to see me grow up but who I hope would be proud of me and thrilled to know their early love and devotion helped pave the way for my beautiful and blessed life.

References

Introduction

1   https://www.huffpost.com/entry/say-goodbye-to-the-girls_b_4829907. Accessed 6/15/22.
2   Latte-Naor S, Mao JJ. Putting Integrative Oncology into Practice: Concepts and Approaches. J Oncol Pract. 2019 Jan;15(1):7-14.
3   https://cancercontrol.cancer.gov/overview-highlights/2021/progress_ocs.html. Accessed 6/15/22.
4   Corner, Jessica. Addressing the needs of cancer survivors: issues and challenges. Expert Review of Pharmacoeconomics & Outcomes Research. 2008; 8:5, 443-451.

Chapter 2: How to Talk So Your Oncologist Listens, and Listen So Your Oncologist Talks

5   Tattersall, Martin H.N. Patient-Oncologist Communication: Sharing Decisions in Cancer Care. Journal of Oncology Practice 2018 14:1, 9-10.
6   Alpert JM, Morris BB, Thomson MD, Matin K, Brown RF. Implications of Patient Portal Transparency in Oncology: Qualitative Interview Study on the Experiences of Patients, Oncologists, and Medical Informaticists. JMIR Cancer. 2018; 4(1):e5.
7   Translational Medicine. https://en.wikipedia.org/wiki/Translational_medicine. Accessed 6/15/22.
8   Shanmugam MK, Rane G, Kanchi MM, Arfuso F, Chinnathambi et al. The multifaceted role of curcumin in cancer prevention and treatment. Molecules. 2015 Feb 5;20(2):2728-69.
9   Oncology Association of Naturopathic Physicians. https://oncanp.org. Accessed 6/15/22.
10 Beers E, Lee Nilsen M, Johnson JT. The Role of Patients: Shared Decision-Making. Otolaryngol Clin North Am. 2017 Aug;50(4):689-708.

11   Farber, A. Mazlich, E. How to Talk So Kids Listen and Listen So Kids Talk. New York, New York: Scribner; 2012.

Chapter 3: Naturopathic Medicine Explained

12   Rothenberg, Amy. The A Cappella Singer Who Lost Her Voice and Other Stories from Natural Medicine. BJain Publishers 2010. Reprinted New England School of Homeopathy Press. 2022.

13   Finnell JS, Snider P, Myers SP, Zeff J. A Hierarchy of Healing: Origins of the Therapeutic Order and Implications for Research. Integr Med. 2019 Jun;18(3):54-59.

14   Fleming SA, Gutknecht NC. Naturopathy and the primary care practice. Prim Care. 2010 Mar;37(1):119-36.

15   Marsden E, Nigh G, Birdsall S, Wright H, Traub M. Oncology Association of Naturopathic Physicians: Principles of Care Guidelines. Curr Oncol. 2019 Feb;26(1):12-18.

Chapter 4: Macroenvironment, Microenvironment, and the Microbiome

16   MD Anderson Cancer Center. What is the Tumor Microenviroment-3 Things to Know. https://www.mdanderson.org/cancerwise/what-is-the-tumor-microenvironment-3-things-to-know.h00-159460056.html. Accessed 6/15/22.

17   Ibid.

18   Arneth B. Tumor Microenvironment. Medicina (Kaunas). 2019 Dec 30;56(1):15.

19   Sanegre S, Lucantoni F, Burgos-Panadero R, et al. Integrating the Tumor Microenvironment into Cancer Therapy. Cancers (Basel). 2020 Jun 24;12(6):1677.

20   Chan-Ran Park, Jin-Seok Lee, Chang-Gue Son, Nam-Hun Lee. A survey of herbal medicines as tumor microenvironment-modulating agents. 2020. Phytotherapy Research 35;1. Pages: 78-94.

21   Lenzi M, Fimognari C, Hrelia P. Sulforaphane as a promising molecule for fighting cancer. Cancer Treat Res. 2014;159:207-23.

22   Zhang L, Zhang H, Li X, Li W, Wang S, Cho CH, Shen J, Li M. Repurposing vitamin D for treatment of human malignancies via targeting tumor microenvironment. Acta Pharm Sin B. 2019 Mar;9(2):203-219.

23   Shreiner AB, Kao JY, Young VB. The gut microbiome in health and in disease. Curr Opin Gastroenterol. 2015 Jan;31(1):69-75.

24   Yuhao Wang et.al. The intestinal microbiota regulates body composition through NFIL 3 and the circadian clock. Science. 2017 Sept 1, Vol 357; 912-916.

25   Zheng D, Liwinski T, Elinav E. Interaction between microbiota and immunity in health and disease. Cell Res. 2020 Jun;30(6):492-506.

26   Guven DC, Aktas BY, Simsek C, Aksoy S. Gut microbiota and cancer immunotherapy: prognostic and therapeutic implications. Future Oncol. 2020 Mar;16(9):497-506.

27   Weiss GA, Hennet T. Mechanisms and consequences of intestinal dysbiosis. Cell Mol Life Sci. 2017 Aug;74(16):2959-2977.

28   Conlon MA, Bird AR. The impact of diet and lifestyle on gut microbiota and human health. Nutrients. 2014 Dec 24;7(1):17-44.

29   Molina-Torres G, Rodriguez-Arrastia M, Roman P, Sanchez-Labraca N, Cardona D. Stress and the gut microbiota-brain axis. Behav Pharmacol. 2019 Apr;30(2 and 3-Spec Issue):187-200.

30   Caitlin A. Selway, et. Al. Transfer of environmental microbes to the skin and respiratory tract of humans after urban green space exposure. Environment International, Volume 145, 2020.

31   Hill C, Guarner F, et al. Expert consensus document. The International Scientific Association for Probiotics and Prebiotics consensus statement on the scope and appropriate use of the term probiotic. Nat Rev Gastroenterol Hepatol. 2014. Aug;11(8):506-14.

32   Doron S, Snydman DR. Risk and safety of probiotics. Clin Infect Dis. 2015 May 15;60 Suppl 2(Suppl 2):S129-34.

33   Davani-Davari D, et al. Prebiotics: Definition, Types, Sources, Mechanisms, and Clinical Applications. Foods. 2019 Mar 9;8(3):92.

34   Thiruvengadam M, et.al. Emerging role of nutritional short-chain fatty acids (SCFAs) against cancer via modulation of hematopoiesis. Crit Rev Food Sci Nutr. 2021 Jul 28:1-18.

Chapter 5: Exercise, Your New Best Friend

35   Garcia DO, Thomson CA. Physical activity and cancer survivorship. Nutr Clin Pract. 2014 Dec;29(6):768-79.

36   Ferrer RA, Huedo-Medina TB, Johnson BT, Ryan S, Pescatello LS. Exercise interventions for cancer survivors: a meta-analysis of quality of life outcomes. Ann Behav Med. 2011 Feb;41(1):32-47.

37   LaVoy EC, Fagundes CP, Dantzer R. Exercise, inflammation, and fatigue in cancer survivors. Exerc Immunol Rev. 2016;22:82-93.

38   Strasser B, Steindorf K, Wiskemann J, Ulrich CM. Impact of resistance training in cancer survivors: a meta-analysis. Med Sci Sports Exerc. 2013 Nov;45(11):2080-90.

39   Almstedt HC, Grote S, Korte JR, et al. Combined aerobic and resistance training improves bone health of female cancer survivors. Bone Rep. 2016 Sep 21;5:274-279.

40   Howden EJ, Bigaran A, Beaudry R, et al. Exercise as a diagnostic and therapeutic tool for the prevention of cardiovascular dysfunction in breast cancer patients. Eur J Prev Cardiol. 2019 Feb;26(3):305-315.

41   Qiaoyun Wang, Wenli Zhou, Roles and molecular mechanisms of physical exercise in cancer prevention and treatment. Journal of Sport and Health Science. 2021; 201-210.

42   van Doorslaer de Ten Ryen S, Deldicque L. The Regulation of the Metastatic Cascade by Physical Activity: A Narrative Review. Cancers (Basel). 2020 Jan 8;12(1):153.

43   Lopes JSS, Machado AF, Micheletti JK, de Almeida AC, Cavina AP, Pastre CM. Effects of training with elastic resistance versus conventional resistance on muscular strength: A systematic review and meta-analysis. SAGE Open Med. 2019 Feb; 19;7.

44   Agarwal RP, Maroko-Afek A. Yoga into Cancer Care: A Review of Evidence-based Research. Int J Yoga. 2018 Jan-Apr;11(1):3-29.

45   How Ballroom Dance Makes Me a Better Doctor https://www.huffpost.com/entry/how-ballroom-dance-makes-_b_6104284. Accessed 6/15/22.

Chapter 6: Diet and Nutrition, Intermittent Fasting, and Reaching Optimal Weight

46   American Cancer Society Guidelines on Nutrition and Physical Activity. The American Cancer Society. https://www.cancer.org/healthy/eat-healthy-get-active/acs-guidelines-nutrition-physical-activity-cancer-prevention/guidelines. Accessed 6/15/22.

47   Weber DD, Aminazdeh-Gohari S, Kofler B. Ketogenic diet in cancer therapy. Aging. 2018 Feb 11;10(2):164-165.

48   What Advanced Training do Naturopathic Doctors Receive? The Institute for Natural Medicine. https://naturemed.org/faq/faq-what-advanced-nutrition-training-do-naturopathic-doctors-receive/. Accessed 6/15/22.

49   Eiró N, Vizoso FJ. Inflammation and cancer. World J Gastrointest Surg. 2012 Mar 27;4(3):62-72.

50   Leenders M, Siersema PD, Overvad K, et al. Subtypes of fruit and vegetables, variety in consumption and risk of colon and rectal cancer in the European Prospective Investigation into Cancer and Nutrition. Int J Cancer. 2015 Dec 1;137(11):2705-14.

51   Alcohol and Cancer Risk. National Cancer Institute. https://www. cancer.gov/about-cancer/causes-prevention/risk/alcohol/alcohol-fact-sheet Accessed 6/15/22.

52   Bultman SJ. Emerging roles of the microbiome in cancer. Carcinogenesis. 2014 Feb;35(2):249-55.

53   Meyerhardt JA, Sato K, Niedzwiecki D, et al. Dietary glycemic load and cancer recurrence and survival in patients with stage III colon cancer: findings from CALGB 89803. J Natl Cancer Inst. 2012 Nov 21;104(22):1702-11.

54   Maskarinec G. Cancer protective properties of cocoa: a review of the epidemiologic evidence. Nutr Cancer. 2009;61(5):573-9.

55   Stoner GD. Foodstuffs for preventing cancer: the preclinical and clinical development of berries. Cancer Prev Res (Phila). 2009 Mar;2(3):187-94.

56   Zhou K, Raffoul JJ. Potential anticancer properties of grape antioxidants. J Oncol. 2012;2012:803294.

57   Aune D, Keum N, Giovannucci E, et al. Nut consumption and risk of cardiovascular disease, total cancer, all-cause and cause-specific mortality: a systematic review and dose-response meta-analysis of prospective studies. BMC Med. 2016 Dec 5;14(1):207.

58   Lima A, Oliveira J, Saúde F et al. Proteins in Soy Might Have a Higher Role in Cancer Prevention than Previously Expected: Soybean Protein Fractions Are More Effective MMP-9 Inhibitors Than Non-Protein Fractions, Even in Cooked Seeds. Nutrients. 2017 Feb 27;9(3):201.

59   Gorzynik-Debicka M, Przychodzen P, Cappello F, et al. Potential Health Benefits of Olive Oil and Plant Polyphenols. Int J Mol Sci. 2018 Feb 28;19(3):686.

60   Syed DN, Chamcheu JC, Adhami VM, Mukhtar H. Pomegranate extracts and cancer prevention: molecular and cellular activities. Anticancer Agents Med Chem. 2013 Oct;13(8):1149-61.

61   Fujiki H, Watanabe T, Sueoka E, et al. Cancer Prevention with Green Tea and Its Principal Constituent, EGCG: from Early Investigations to Current Focus on Human Cancer Stem Cells. Mol Cells. 2018 Feb 28;41(2):73-82.

62   Goyal A, Sharma V, Upadhyay N. et al. Flax and flaxseed oil: an ancient medicine & modern functional food. J Food Sci Technol. 2014 Sep;51(9):1633-53.

63   Baliga MS, Haniadka R, Pereira MM, et al. Update on the chemopreventive effects of ginger and its phytochemicals. Crit Rev Food Sci Nutr. 2011 Jul;51(6):499-523.

64   Park W, Amin AR, Chen ZG, Shin DM. New perspectives of curcumin in cancer prevention. Cancer Prev Res (Phila). 2013 May;6(5):387-400.

65   Nicastro HL, Ross SA, Milner JA. Garlic and onions: their cancer prevention properties. Cancer Prev Res (Phila). 2015 Mar;8(3):181-9.

66   Sadeghi S, Davoodvandi A, Pourhanifeh MH, et al. Anti-cancer effects of cinnamon: Insights into its apoptosis effects. Eur J Med Chem. 2019 Sep 15;178:131-140.

67   Patel S, Goyal A. Recent developments in mushrooms as anti-cancer therapeutics: a review. Biotech. 2012 Mar;2(1):1-15.

68   Farvid MS, Spence ND, Rosner BA, Willett WC, Eliassen AH, Holmes MD. Post-diagnostic coffee and tea consumption and breast cancer survival. Br J Cancer. 2021;124(11):1873-1881.

69   The carcinogenicity of the consumption of red meat and processed meat. The World Health Organization. https://www.who.int/news-room/q-a-detail/cancer-carcinogenicity-of-the-consumption-of-red-meat-and-processed-meat. Accessed 6/15/22.

70   D'Elia L, Galletti F, Strazzullo P. Dietary salt intake and risk of gastric cancer. Cancer Treat Res. 2014;159:83-95.

71   Recipes from Dr. Rothenberg. https://dramyrothenberg.com/resources/recipes/. Accessed 6/15/22.

72   Mattson MP, Longo VD, Harvie M. Impact of intermittent fasting on health and disease processes. Ageing Res Rev. 2017 Oct;39:46-58.

73   Marinac CR, Nelson SH, Breen CI, et al. Prolonged Nightly Fasting and Breast Cancer Prognosis. JAMA Oncol. 2016 Aug 1;2(8):1049-55.

74   Alirezaei M, Kemball CC, Flynn CT, et al. Short-term fasting induces profound neuronal autophagy. Autophagy. 2010 Aug;6(6):702-10.

75   Nencioni A, Caffa I, Cortellino S, Longo VD. Fasting and cancer: molecular mechanisms and clinical application. Nat Rev Cancer. 2018 Nov;18(11):707-719.

76   Calle EE, Rodriguez C, Walker-Thurmond K, Thun MJ. Overweight, obesity, and mortality from cancer in a prospectively studied cohort of U.S. adults. N Engl J Med. 2003 Apr 24;348(17):1625-38.

77   State of Obesity 2020. The Trust for America's Health. https://www.tfah.org/report-details/state-of-obesity-2020/ Accessed 6/15/22.

78   Varady KA, Cienfuegos S, Ezpeleta M, Gabel K. Cardiometabolic Benefits of Intermittent Fasting. Annu Rev Nutr. 2021 Oct 11;41:333-361.

79   Aoun A, Darwish F, Hamod N. The Influence of the Gut Microbiome on Obesity in Adults and the Role of Probiotics, Prebiotics, and Synbiotics for Weight Loss. Prev Nutr Food Sci. 2020 Jun 30;25(2):113-123.

80   Kunduraci YE, Ozbek H. Does the Energy Restriction Intermittent Fasting Diet Alleviate Metabolic Syndrome Biomarkers? A Randomized Controlled Trial. Nutrients. 2020 Oct 21;12(10):3213.

81   Janesick AS, Blumberg B. Obesogens: an emerging threat to public health. Am J Obstet Gynecol. 2016 May;214(5):559-65.

82   Diamanti-Kandarakis E, Bourguignon JP, Giudice LC, et al. Endocrine-disrupting chemicals: an Endocrine Society scientific statement. Endocr Rev. 2009 Jun;30(4):293-342.

83   Griffin MD, Pereira SR, DeBari MK, Abbott RD. Mechanisms of action, chemical characteristics, and model systems of obesogens. BMC Biomed Eng. 2020 Apr 30;2:6.

84   Heindel JJ, Vom Saal FS, Blumberg B, et al. Parma consensus statement on metabolic disruptors. Environ Health. 2015 Jun 20;14:54.

Chapter 7: Nutritional Supplements

85   Hamzehzadeh L, Atkin SL, Majeed M, Butler AE, Sahebkar A. The versatile role of curcumin in cancer prevention and treatment: A focus on PI3K/AKT pathway. J Cell Physiol. 2018 Oct;233(10):6530-6537.

86   Khan N, Mukhtar H. Cancer and metastasis: prevention and treatment by green tea. Cancer Metastasis Rev. 2010 Sep;29(3):435-45.

87   Patel S, Goyal A. Recent developments in mushrooms as anti-cancer therapeutics: a review. Biotech. 2012 Mar;2(1):1-15.

88   Ibid.

89   Nam JS, Sharma AR, Nguyen LT, Chakraborty C, Sharma G, Lee SS. Application of Bioactive Quercetin in Oncotherapy: From Nutrition to Nanomedicine. Molecules. 2016 Jan 19;21(1):E108.

90   Reiter RJ, Rosales-Corral SA, Tan DX, et al. Melatonin, a Full Service Anti-Cancer Agent: Inhibition of Initiation, Progression and Metastasis. Int J Mol Sci. 2017 Apr 17;18(4):843.

91   Elshaer M, Chen Y, Wang XJ, Tang X. Resveratrol: An overview of its anti-cancer mechanisms. Life Sci. 2018 Aug 15;207:340-349.

92   Salehi B, Berkay Yılmaz Y, Antika G. Insights on the Use of α-Lipoic Acid for Therapeutic Purposes. Biomolecules. 2019 Aug 9;9(8):356.

93   Garland CF, Garland FC, Gorham ED, et al. The role of vitamin D in cancer prevention. Am J Public Health. 2006 Feb;96(2):252-61.

94   Nabavi SF, Bilotto S, Russo GL, et al. Omega-3 polyunsaturated fatty acids and cancer: lessons learned from clinical trials. Cancer Metastasis Rev. 2015 Sep;34(3):359-80.

95   Du M, Luo H, Blumberg JB, et al. Dietary Supplement Use among Adult Cancer Survivors in the United States. J Nutr. 2020 Jun 1;150(6):1499-1508.

Chapter 8: Botanical Medicine

96   Petrovic V, Nepal A, Olaisen C, et al. Anti-Cancer Potential of Homemade Fresh Garlic Extract Is Related to Increased Endoplasmic Reticulum Stress. Nutrients. 2018 Apr 5;10(4):450.

97 Kujundžić RN, Stepanić V, Milković L, et al. Curcumin and its Potential for Systemic Targeting of Inflamm-Aging and Metabolic Reprogramming in Cancer. Int J Mol Sci. 2019 Mar 8;20(5):1180.

98 De Lima RMT, Dos Reis AC, de Menezes APM, et al. Protective and therapeutic potential of ginger (Zingiber officinale) extract and [6]-gingerol in cancer: A comprehensive review. Phytother Res. 2018 Oct;32(10):1885-1907.

99 Blagodatski A, Yatsunskaya M, Mikhailova V, et al. Medicinal mushrooms as an attractive new source of natural compounds for future cancer therapy. Oncotarget. 2018 Jun 26;9(49):29259-29274.

100 Ortiz LM, Lombardi P, Tillhon M, Scovassi AI. Berberine, an epiphany against cancer. Molecules. 2014 Aug 15;19(8):12349-67.

101 Auyeung KK, Han QB, Ko JK. Astragalus membranaceus: A Review of its Protection Against Inflammation and Gastrointestinal Cancers. Am J Chin Med. 2016;44(1):1-22.

102 Fujiki H, Watanabe T, Sueoka E, Rawangkan A, Suganuma M. Cancer Prevention with Green Tea and Its Principal Constituent, EGCG: from Early Investigations to Current Focus on Human Cancer Stem Cells. Mol Cells. 2018 Feb 28;41(2):73-82.

103 Vervandier-Fasseur D, Latruffe N. The Potential Use of Resveratrol for Cancer Prevention. Molecules. 2019 Dec 9;24(24):4506.

104 Jin X, Che DB, Zhang ZH, Yan HM, Jia ZY, Jia XB. Ginseng consumption and risk of cancer: A meta-analysis. J Ginseng Res. 2016 Jul;40(3):269-77.

105 Yan Xie, Benjamin Bowe, Tingting Li, Hong Xian, Yan Yan, Ziyad Al-Aly. Risk of death among users of Proton Pump Inhibitors: a longitudinal observational cohort study of United States veterans. BMJ Open, 2017; 7 (6): e015735.

106 Yeh AM, Golianu B. Integrative Treatment of Reflux and Functional Dyspepsia in Children. Children (Basel). 2014 Aug 18;1(2):119-33.

107 Panahi Y, Khedmat H, Valizadegan G, Mohtashami R, Sahebkar A. Efficacy and safety of Aloe vera syrup for the treatment of gastro-esophageal reflux disease: a pilot randomized positive-controlled trial. J Tradit Chin Med. 2015 Dec;35(6):632-6.

108 Andersen BN, Johansen PB, Abrahamsen B. Proton pump inhibitors and osteoporosis. Curr Opin Rheumatol. 2016 Jul;28(4):420-5

109 Yibirin M, De Oliveira D, Valera R, Plitt AE, Lutgen S. Adverse Effects Associated with Proton Pump Inhibitor Use. Cureus. 2021 Jan 18;13(1):e12759.

110 Lillehei AS, Halcón LL, Savik K, Reis R. Effect of Inhaled Lavender and Sleep Hygiene on Self-Reported Sleep Issues: A Randomized Controlled Trial. J Altern Complement Med. 2015 Jul;21(7):430-8.

111   Yeung KS, Hernandez M, Mao JJ, Haviland I, Gubili J. Herbal medicine for depression and anxiety: A systematic review with assessment of potential psycho-oncologic relevance. Phytother Res. 2018 May;32(5):865-891.

112   Tiralongo E, Wee SS, Lea RA. Elderberry Supplementation Reduces Cold Duration and Symptoms in Air-Travellers: A Randomized, Double-Blind Placebo-Controlled Clinical Trial. Nutrients. 2016 Mar 24;8(4):182.

113   Sengupta K, Alluri KV, Satish AR, et al. A double blind, randomized, placebo controlled study of the efficacy and safety of 5-Loxin for treatment of osteoarthritis of the knee. Arthritis Res Ther. 2008;10(4):R85.

114   Akaberi M, Sahebkar A, Emami SA. Turmeric and Curcumin: From Traditional to Modern Medicine. Adv Exp Med Biol. 2021;1291:15-39.

Chapter 9: Whole-Person Medicines: Homeopathy/ Acupuncture

115   Fixsen A. Homeopathy in the Age of Antimicrobial Resistance: Is It a Viable Treatment for Upper Respiratory Tract Infections? Homeopathy. 2018 May;107(2):99-114.

116   Zanasi A, Mazzolini M, Tursi F, Morselli-Labate AM, Paccapelo A, Lecchi M. Homeopathic medicine for acute cough in upper respiratory tract infections and acute bronchitis: a randomized, double-blind, placebo-controlled trial. Pulm Pharmacol Ther. 2014 Feb;27(1):102-8.

117   Ventola CL. The antibiotic resistance crisis: part 1: causes and threats. PT. 2015 Apr;40(4):277-83.

118   Weidong Lu, David S. Rosenthal, Oncology Acupuncture for Chronic Pain in Cancer Survivors: A Reflection on the American Society of Clinical Oncology Chronic Pain Guideline, Hematology/Oncology Clinics of North America, Volume 32, Issue 3, 2018, Pages 519-533.

119   Li H, Schlaeger JM, Jang MK, et al.Acupuncture Improves Multiple Treatment-Related Symptoms in Breast Cancer Survivors: A Systematic Review and Meta-Analysis. J Altern Complement Med. 2021 Aug 27.

120   Spence DS, Thompson EA, Barron SJ. Homeopathic treatment for chronic disease: a 6-year, university-hospital outpatient observational study. J Altern Complement Med. 2005 Oct;11(5):793-8.

121   Vickers, Andrew J. et al. Acupuncture for Chronic Pain: Update of an Individual Patient Data Meta-Analysis. The Journal of Pain, Volume 19, Issue 5, 455–474.

122   Birch, Stephen. Treating the patient not the symptoms: Acupuncture to improve overall health – Evidence, acceptance and strategies. Integrative Medicine Research, Volume 8, Issue 1, 2019, Pages 33-41.

Chapter 10: Using Prescribed Medication Alongside Natural Medicine and the Off-Label Use of Pharmaceuticals

123   Hales CM, Servais J, Martin CB, Kohen D. Prescription Drug Use Among Adults Aged 40-79 in the United States and Canada. NCHS Data Brief. 2019 Aug;(347):1-8.

124   2019 AGS Beers Criteria for older adults. American Pharmacist Association. https://www.pharmacytoday.org/article/S1042-0991(19)31235-6/pdf Accessed 6/15/22.

125   AGS Beers Criteria Pocket Card. American Geriatric Association. https://www.elderconsult.com/wp-content/uploads/PrintableBeersPocketCard.pdf Accessed 6/15/22.

126   Meyers RS, Thackray J, Matson KL, et al. Key Potentially Inappropriate Drugs in Pediatrics: The KIDs List. J Pediatr Pharmacol Ther. 2020;25(3):175-191.

127   Scott IA, Hilmer SN, Reeve E, et al. Reducing inappropriate polypharmacy: the process of deprescribing. JAMA Intern Med. 2015 May;175(5):827-34.

128   FAQ Series on Common Health Complaints. Institute for Natural Medicine Website: https://naturemed.org. Accessed 6/15/22.

129   Jin Y, Desta Z, Stearns V, et al. CYP2D6 genotype, antidepressant use, and tamoxifen metabolism during adjuvant breast cancer treatment. J Natl Cancer Inst. 2005 Jan 5;97(1):30-9.

130   Probability of success for oncology vs non-oncology drugs in the U.S. in the different development phases from 2011 to 2020. Statista. https://www.statista.com/statistics/597819/drug-development-phases-probability-of-success-oncology-nononcology-drugs/ Accessed 6/15/22.

131   Pantziarka P, Bouche G, Meheus L, et al. The Repurposing Drugs in Oncology (ReDO) Project. Ecancermedicalscience. 2014 Jul 10;8:442.

132   Yin M, Zhou J, Gorak EJ, Quddus F. Metformin is associated with survival benefit in cancer patients with concurrent type 2 diabetes: a systematic review and meta-analysis. Oncologist. 2013;18(12):1248-55.

133   Listing of clinical trial related to Metformin and Cancer. The National Institute of Health. https://www.clinicaltrials.gov/ct2/results?term=metformin+and+cancer&Search=Search Accessed 6/15/22.

134   Del Barco S, Vazquez-Martin A, Cufí S, Metformin: multi-faceted protection against cancer. Oncotarget. 2011 Dec;2(12):896-917.

135   Wang H, Zhu C, Ying Y, et al. Metformin and berberine, two versatile drugs in treatment of common metabolic diseases. Oncotarget. 2017 Sep 11;9(11):10135-10146.

136 Spugnini E, Fais S. Proton pump inhibition and cancer therapeutics: A specific tumor targeting or it is a phenomenon secondary to a systemic buffering? Semin Cancer Biol. 2017 Apr;43:111-118.

137 Mills EJ, Wu P, Alberton M, Kanters S, Lanas A, Lester R. Low-dose aspirin and cancer mortality: a meta-analysis of randomized trials. Am J Med. 2012 Jun;125(6):560-7.

138 Pantziarka P, Verbaanderd C, Sukhatme V, ReDO_DB: the repurposing drugs in oncology database. Ecancermedicalscience. 2018 Dec 6;12:886.

139 Ibid.

Chapter 11: The Head Game, Stress, and Stress Reduction

140 Nagoski, Amelia, Nagoski, Emily. Burnout-The Secret to Unlocking the Stress Cycle. New York, New York. Random House Publishing Group. 2021.

141 Jeon SW, Kim YK. Inflammation-induced depression: Its pathophysiology and therapeutic implications. J Neuroimmunol. 2017 Dec 15;313:92-98.

142 Seo JS, Wei J, Qin L, Kim Y, Yan Z, Greengard P. Cellular and molecular basis for stress-induced depression. Mol Psychiatry. 2017 Oct;22(10):1440-1447.

143 Dauchy S, Dolbeault S, Reich M. Depression in cancer patients. EJC Suppl. 2013 Sep;11(2):205-15.

144 Satin JR, Linden W, Phillips MJ. Depression as a predictor of disease progression and mortality in cancer patients: a meta-analysis. Cancer. 2009 Nov 15;115(22):5349-61.

145 Ostuzzi G, Matcham F, Dauchy S, Barbui C, Hotopf M. Antidepressants for the treatment of depression in people with cancer. Cochrane Database Syst Rev. 2018 Apr 23;4(4).

146 Mir O, Durand JP, Boudou-Rouquette P, et al. Interaction between serotonin reuptake inhibitors, 5-HT3 antagonists, and NK1 antagonists in cancer patients receiving highly emetogenic chemotherapy: a case-control study. Support Care Cancer. 2012 Sep;20(9):2235-9.

147 Christensen DK, Armaiz-Pena GN, Ramirez E, et al. SSRI use and clinical outcomes in epithelial ovarian cancer. Oncotarget. 2016 May 31;7(22):33179-91.

148 Raman-Wilms L, Farrell B, Sadowski C, Austin Z. Deprescribing: An educational imperative. Res Social Adm Pharm. 2019 Jun;15(6):790-795.

149 Cipolletta S, Simonato C, Faccio E. The Effectiveness of Psychoeducational Support Groups for Women With Breast Cancer and Their Caregivers: A Mixed Methods Study. Front Psychol. 2019 Feb 18;10:288.

150   Cramer H, Lauche R, Klose P, Lange S, Langhorst J, Dobos GJ. Yoga for improving health-related quality of life, mental health and cancer-related symptoms in women diagnosed with breast cancer. Cochrane Database Syst Rev. 2017 Jan 3;1.

151   Johnson JA, Rash JA, Campbell TS, et al. A systematic review and meta-analysis of randomized controlled trials of cognitive behavior therapy for insomnia (CBT-I) in cancer survivors. Sleep Med Rev. 2016 Jun;27:20-8.

152   Ye M, Du K, Zhou J, et al. A meta-analysis of the efficacy of cognitive behavior therapy on quality of life and psychological health of breast cancer survivors and patients. Psychooncology. 2018 Jul;27(7):1695-1703.

153   Tala Á. Gracias por todo: Una revisión sobre la gratitud desde la neurobiología a la clínica [Thanks for everything: a review on gratitude from neurobiology to clinic]. Rev Med Chil. 2019 Jun;147(6):755-761. Spanish.

154   Gary H. Lyman, Heather Greenlee, Kari Bohlke, et al. Integrative Therapies During and After Breast Cancer Treatment: ASCO Endorsement of the SIO Clinical Practice Guidelines. Journal of Clinical Oncology 2018 36:25, 2647-2655.

155   Limbana T, Khan F, Eskander N. Gut Microbiome and Depression: How Microbes Affect the Way We Think. Cureus. 2020 Aug 23;12(8):e9966.

156   Packard AE, Egan AE, Ulrich-Lai YM. HPA Axis Interactions with Behavioral Systems. Compr Physiol. 2016 Sep 15;6(4):1897-193.

157   Nuss P. Anxiety disorders and GABA neurotransmission: a disturbance of modulation. Neuropsychiatr Dis Treat. 2015 Jan 17;11:165-75.

158   White DJ, de Klerk S, Woods W, Gondalia S, Noonan C, Scholey AB. Anti-Stress, Behavioural and Magnetoencephalography Effects of an L-Theanine-Based Nutrient Drink: A Randomised, Double-Blind, Placebo-Controlled, Crossover Trial. Nutrients. 2016 Jan 19;8(1):53.

159   Post RM. The New News about Lithium: An Underutilized Treatment in the United States. Neuropsychopharmacology. 2018 Apr;43(5):1174-1179.

160   Wang J, Um P, Dickerman BA, Liu J. Zinc, Magnesium, Selenium and Depression: A Review of the Evidence, Potential Mechanisms and Implications. Nutrients. 2018 May 9;10(5):584.

161   28Apaydin EA, et al. A systematic review of St. John's wort for major depressive disorder. Syst Rev. 2016 Sep 2;5(1):148. doi: 10.1186/s13643-016-0325-2. PMID: 27589952; PMCID: PMC5010734.

162   Ng QX, Koh SSH, Chan HW, Ho CYX. Clinical Use of Curcumin in Depression: A Meta-Analysis. J Am Med Dir Assoc. 2017 Jun 1;18(6):503-508.

163 Shafiee M, Arekhi S, Omranzadeh A, Sahebkar A. Saffron in the treatment of depression, anxiety and other mental disorders: Current evidence and potential mechanisms of action. J Affect Disord. 2018 Feb;227:330-337.

164 Lewis JE, et al. The effect of methylated vitamin B complex on depressive and anxiety symptoms and quality of life in adults with depression. ISRN Psychiatry. 2013 Jan 21;2013:621453.

165 Burhani MD, Rasenick MM. Fish oil and depression: The skinny on fats. J Integr Neurosci. 2017;16(s1):S115-S124.

166 Maffei ME. 5-Hydroxytryptophan (5-HTP): Natural Occurrence, Analysis, Biosynthesis, Biotechnology, Physiology and Toxicology. Int J Mol Sci. 2020 Dec 26;22(1):181.

167 Lopresti AL, Smith SJ, Malvi H, Kodgule R. An investigation into the stress-relieving and pharmacological actions of an ashwagandha (Withania somnifera) extract: A randomized, double-blind, placebo-controlled study. Medicine (Baltimore). 2019 Sep;98(37):e17186.

168 da Fonseca LR, Rodrigues RA, Ramos AS, et al. Herbal Medicinal Products from Passiflora for Anxiety: An Unexploited Potential. ScientificWorldJournal. 2020 Jul 20;2020:6598434.

169 Koulivand PH, Khaleghi Ghadiri M, Gorji A. Lavender and the nervous system. Evid Based Complement Alternat Med. 2013;2013:681304.

170 25 Melrose S. Seasonal Affective Disorder: An Overview of Assessment and Treatment Approaches. Depress Res Treat. 2015;2015:178564.

171 Virk G, Reeves G, Rosenthal NE, Sher L, Postolache TT. Short exposure to light treatment improves depression scores in patients with seasonal affective disorder: A brief report. Int J Disabil Hum Dev. 2009 Jul;8(3):283-286.

172 Sarkar, S. Vitamin D for depression with a seasonal pattern: an effective treatment strategy. International Physical Medicine and Rehabilitation Journal. Volume 1, issue 4. 2017.

Chapter 12: Get Your Rest!

173 Sara E. Strollo, Elizabeth A. Fallon, Susan M. Gapstur, Tenbroeck G. Smith, Cancer-related problems, sleep quality, and sleep disturbance among long-term cancer survivors at 9-years post diagnosis, Sleep Medicine. Volume 65, 2020, Pages 177-185.

174 Brudnowska J, Pepłońska B. Praca zmianowa nocna a ryzyko choroby nowotworowej—przeglad literatury [Night shift work and cancer risk: a literature review]. Med Pr. 2011;62(3):323-38.

175 In U.S., 40% Get Less Than Recommended Amount of Sleep. Gallup. https://news.gallup.com/poll/166553/less-recommended-amount-sleep.aspx. Accessed 6/15/22.

176 Lydiard RB. The role of GABA in anxiety disorders. J Clin Psychiatry. 2003;64 Suppl 3:21-7.

177 Lu K, Gray MA, Oliver C, et al. The acute effects of L-theanine in comparison with alprazolam on anticipatory anxiety in humans. Hum Psychopharmacol. 2004 Oct;19(7):457-65.

178 Chen WY, Giobbie-Hurder A, Gantman K, et al. A randomized, placebo-controlled trial of melatonin on breast cancer survivors: impact on sleep, mood, and hot flashes. Breast Cancer Res Treat. 2014 Jun;145(2):381-8.

179 Talib WH, Alsayed AR, Abuawad A, Daoud S, Mahmod AI. Melatonin in Cancer Treatment: Current Knowledge and Future Opportunities. Molecules. 2021 Apr 25;26(9):2506.

180 Akhondzadeh S, Naghavi HR, Vazirian M, Shayeganpour A, Rashidi H, Khani M. Passionflower in the treatment of generalized anxiety: a pilot double-blind randomized controlled trial with oxazepam. J Clin Pharm Ther. 2001 Oct;26(5):363-7.

181 Koetter U, Schrader E, Käufeler R, Brattström A. A randomized, double blind, placebo-controlled, prospective clinical study to demonstrate clinical efficacy of a fixed valerian hops extract combination (Ze 91019) in patients suffering from non-organic sleep disorder. Phytother Res. 2007 Sep;21(9):847-51.

182 Kaushik MK, Kaul SC, Wadhwa R, Yanagisawa M, Urade Y. Triethylene glycol, an active component of Ashwagandha (Withania somnifera) leaves, is responsible for sleep induction. PloS One. 2017 Feb 16;12(2):e0172508.

183 Ferracioli-Oda E, Qawasmi A, Bloch MH. Meta-analysis: melatonin for the treatment of primary sleep disorders. PLoS One. 2013 May 17;8(5):e63773.

184 Kawai N, Sakai N, Okuro M, et al. The sleep-promoting and hypothermic effects of glycine are mediated by NMDA receptors in the suprachiasmatic nucleus. Neuropsychopharmacology. 2015 May;40(6):1405-16.

185 Silber BY, Schmitt JA. Effects of tryptophan loading on human cognition, mood, and sleep. Neurosci Biobehav Rev. 2010 Mar;34(3):387-407.

Chapter 13: Hands-On Bodywork

186 Lee SH, Kim JY, Yeo S, Kim SH, Lim S. Meta-Analysis of Massage Therapy on Cancer Pain. Integr Cancer Ther. 2015 Jul;14(4):297-304.

187 Kinkead B, Schettler PJ, Larson ER, et al. Massage therapy decreases cancer-related fatigue: Results from a randomized early phase trial. Cancer. 2018 Feb 1;124(3):546-554.

188   Lopez G, Liu W, Milbury K, Spelman A, Wei Q, Bruera E, Cohen L. The effects of oncology massage on symptom self-report for cancer patients and their caregivers. Support Care Cancer. 2017 Dec;25(12):3645-3650.

189   Cho Y, Do J, Jung S, Kwon O, Jeon JY. Effects of a physical therapy program combined with manual lymphatic drainage on shoulder function, quality of life, lymphedema incidence, and pain in breast cancer patients with axillary web syndrome following axillary dissection. Support Care Cancer. 2016 May;24(5):2047-2057.

190   Arienti C, Bosisio T, Ratti S, Miglioli R, Negrini S. Osteopathic Manipulative Treatment Effect on Pain Relief and Quality of Life in Oncology Geriatric Patients: A Nonrandomized Controlled Clinical Trial. Integr Cancer Ther. 2018 Dec;17(4):1163-1171.

191   Gonella S, Garrino L, Dimonte V. Biofield therapies and cancer-related symptoms: a review. Clin J Oncol Nurs. 2014 Oct;18(5):568-76.

Chapter 14: Reduce Environmental Toxin Exposure and Support Your Emunctories

192   Cohen L, Jefferies A. Environmental exposures and cancer: using the precautionary principle. Ecancermedicalscience. 2019 Apr 16;13:ed91.

193   National Toxicology Program of the Department of Health and Human Services' 15th Report on Carcinogens. https://ntp.niehs.nih.gov/whatwestudy/assessments/cancer/roc/index.html. Accessed 6/15/22.

194   National Institute of Environmental Health Sciences. Endocrine Disruptors Fact Sheet. https://www.niehs.nih.gov/health/materials/endocrine_disruptors_508.pdf. May 2020. Accessed 6/15/22.

195   Madia F, Worth A, Whelan M, Corvi R. Carcinogenicity assessment: Addressing the challenges of cancer and chemicals in the environment. Environ Int. 2019 Jul;128:417-429.

196   Diamanti-Kandarakis, et al. Endocrine-disrupting chemicals: an Endocrine Society scientific statement. Endocr Rev. 2009 Jun;30(4):293-342.

197   Potera C. Scented products emit a bouquet of VOCs. Environ Health Perspect. 2011 Jan;119(1):A16.

198   Santibáñez-Andrade M, Chirino YI, González-Ramírez, et al. Deciphering the Code between Air Pollution and Disease: The Effect of Particulate Matter on Cancer Hallmarks. Int J Mol Sci. 2019 Dec 24;21(1):136.

199   Brown KW, Gessesse B, Butler LJ, MacIntosh DL. Potential Effectiveness of Point-of-Use Filtration to Address Risks to Drinking Water in the United States. Environ Health Insights. 2017 Dec 12;11:1178630217746997.

200 Center for Disease Control and Prevention. Quit Smoking. https://www.cdc.gov/tobacco/quit_smoking/index.htm. Accessed 6/15/22.

201 Vigar V, Myers S, Oliver C, Arellano J, Robinson S, Leifert C. A Systematic Review of Organic Versus Conventional Food Consumption: Is There a Measurable Benefit on Human Health? Nutrients. 2019 Dec 18;12(1):7.

202 Baudry J, Assmann KE, Touvier M, et al. Association of Frequency of Organic Food Consumption With Cancer Risk: Findings From the NutriNet-Santé Prospective Cohort Study. JAMA Intern Med. 2018 Dec 1;178(12):1597-1606.

203 Myers SP, Kruzel T, Zeff J, Snider P. Emunctorology: Synthesising Traditional Naturopathic Practice with Modern Science. Integr Med (Encinitas). 2019 Jun;18(3):40-41.

204 Crinnion WJ. Sauna as a valuable clinical tool for cardiovascular, auto-immune, toxicant- induced and other chronic health problems. Altern Med Rev. 2011 Sep;16(3):215-25.

Chapter 15: Community and Connection

205 Umberson D, Montez JK. Social relationships and health: a flashpoint for health policy. J Health Soc Behav. 2010;51 Suppl(Suppl):S54-66.

206 Reynolds P, Kaplan GA. Social connections and risk for cancer: prospective evidence from the Alameda County Study. Behav Med.1990 Fall;16(3):101-10.

207 Rogers NT, Demakakos P, Taylor MS, Steptoe A, Hamer M, Shankar A. Volunteering is associated with increased survival in able-bodied participants of the English Longitudinal Study of Ageing. J Epidemiol Community Health. 2016 Jun;70(6):583-8.

208 Namkoong K, Shah DV, Gustafson DH. Offline Social Relationships and Online Cancer Communication: Effects of Social and Family Support on Online Social Network Building. Health Commun. 2017 Nov;32(11):1422-1429.

Chapter 16: Caregivers as Survivors

209 American Rescue Plan by President Joe Biden. https://www.whitehouse.gov/briefing-room/legislation/2021/01/20/president-biden-announces-american-rescue-plan/ Accessed 6/15/22.

210 Caregiving in the United States. American Association of Retired Persons. https://www.aarp.org/content/dam/aarp/ppi/2020/05/full-report-caregiving-in-the-united-states. Retrieved 2/22/22.

211   Hypertension Drugs Recalled Due to Possible Carcinogenic Contaminant, and More to the Point: Naturopathic Approaches to Hypertension. https://tinyurl.com/HighBloodPressureDrRothenberg. Retrieved 3/22/22.

Chapter 17: Naturopathic Recommendations for Specific Health Problems after Cancer Care

212   Baumgart M, Snyder HM, Carrillo MC, Fazio S, Kim H, Johns H. Summary of the evidence on modifiable risk factors for cognitive decline and dementia: A population-based perspective. Alzheimers Dement. 2015 Jun;11(6):718-26.
213   van der Willik KD, Schagen SB, Ikram MA. Cancer and dementia: Two sides of the same coin? Eur J Clin Invest. 2018 Nov;48(11):e13019.
214   Kovalchuk A, Kolb B. Chemo brain: From discerning mechanisms to lifting the brain fog-An aging connection. Cell Cycle. 2017 Jul 18;16(14):1345-1349.
215   Shahid M, Kim J. Exercise May Affect Metabolism in Cancer-Related Cognitive Impairment. Metabolites. 2020 Sep 20;10(9):377.
216   Ahlskog JE, Geda YE, Graff-Radford NR, Petersen RC. Physical exercise as a preventive or disease-modifying treatment of dementia and brain aging. Mayo Clin Proc. 2011 Sep;86(9):876-84.
217   Chin D, Huebbe P, Pallauf K, Rimbach G. Neuroprotective properties of curcumin in Alzheimer's disease--merits and limitations. Curr Med Chem. 2013;20(32):3955-85.
218   Sawda C, Moussa C, Turner RS. Resveratrol for Alzheimer's disease. Ann N Y Acad Sci. 2017 Sep;1403(1):142-149.
219   Aguiar S, Borowski T. Neuropharmacological review of the nootropic herb Bacopa monnieri. Rejuvenation Res. 2013 Aug;16(4):313-26.
220   Loughrey DG, Kelly ME, Kelley GA, Brennan S, Lawlor BA. Association of Age-Related Hearing Loss With Cognitive Function, Cognitive Impairment, and Dementia: A Systematic Review and Meta-analysis. JAMA Otolaryngol Head Neck Surg. 2018 Feb 1;144(2):115-126.
221   Russell-Williams J, Jaroudi W, Perich T, Hoscheidt S, El Haj M, Moustafa AA. Mindfulness and meditation: treating cognitive impairment and reducing stress in dementia. Rev Neurosci. 2018 Sep 25;29(7):791-804.
222   Corsonello A, Lattanzio F, Bustacchini S, et al. Adverse Events of Proton Pump Inhibitors: Potential Mechanisms. Curr Drug Metab. 2018;19(2):142-154.

223   Cheng HT, Lin FJ, Erickson SR, Hong JL, Wu CH. The Association Between the Use of Zolpidem and the Risk of Alzheimer's Disease Among Older People. J Am Geriatr Soc. 2017 Nov;65(11):2488-2495.

Fatigue

224   National Comprehensive Cancer Network. Cancer Related Fatigue. https://oncolife.com.ua/doc/nccn/fatigue.pdf. Accessed 6/15/22.
225   Savina S, Zaydiner B. Cancer-Related Fatigue: Some Clinical Aspects. Asia Pac J Oncol Nurs. 2019 Jan-Mar;6(1):7-9.
226   Dennett AM, Peiris CL, Shields N, Prendergast LA, Taylor NF. Moderate-intensity exercise reduces fatigue and improves mobility in cancer survivors: a systematic review and meta-regression. J Physiother. 2016 Apr;62(2):68-82.
227   Bower JE, Garet D, Sternlieb B, et al. Yoga for persistent fatigue in breast cancer survivors: a randomized controlled trial. Cancer. 2012 Aug 1;118(15):3766-75.
228   Sowada KM. Qigong: Benefits for Survivors Coping with Cancer-Related Fatigue. Clin J Oncol Nurs. 2019 Oct 1;23(5):465-469.
229   Inglis JE, Lin PJ, Kerns SL, et al. Nutritional Interventions for Treating Cancer-Related Fatigue: A Qualitative Review. Nutr Cancer. 2019;71(1):21-40.
230   Capellino, S., Claus, M. & Watzl, C. Regulation of natural killer cell activity by glucocorticoids, serotonin, dopamine, and epinephrine. Cell Mol Immunol 17, 705–711 (2020).
231   https://naturemed.org/are-you-rundown-with-burnout-how-relentless-stress-damages-our-health-and-what-to-do-about-it/ Accessed 6/15/22.
232   Sadeghian M, Rahmani S, Zendehdel M, Hosseini SA, Zare Javid A. Ginseng and Cancer-Related Fatigue: A Systematic Review of Clinical Trials. Nutr Cancer. 2021;73(8):1270-1281.
233   Tardy AL, Pouteau E, Marquez D, Yilmaz C, Scholey A. Vitamins and Minerals for Energy, Fatigue and Cognition: A Narrative Review of the Biochemical and Clinical Evidence. Nutrients. 2020 Jan 16;12(1):228.
234   Ibid.
235   Lopresti AL, Smith SJ, Malvi H, Kodgule R. An investigation into the stress-relieving and pharmacological actions of an ashwagandha (Withania somnifera) extract: A randomized, double-blind, placebo-controlled study. Medicine (Baltimore). 2019 Sep;98(37):e17186.
236   Edwards D, Heufelder A, Zimmermann A. Therapeutic effects and safety of Rhodiola rosea extract WS® 1375 in subjects with life-stress symptoms—results of an open-label study. Phytother Res. 2012 Aug;26(8):1220-5.

237 Yang R, Wang LQ, Yuan BC, Liu Y. The Pharmacological Activities of Licorice. Planta Med. 2015 Dec;81(18):1654-69.

238 Hewlings SJ, Kalman DS. Curcumin: A Review of Its Effects on Human Health. Foods. 2017 Oct 22;6(10):92.

239 Jang A, Brown C, Lamoury G, et al. The Effects of Acupuncture on Cancer-Related Fatigue: Updated Systematic Review and Meta-Analysis. Integr Cancer Ther. 2020 Jan-Dec;19: 1534735420949679

Lack of Interest and/or Satisfaction with Sex

240 Schover LR. Sexual quality of life in men and women after cancer. Climacteric. 2019 Dec;22(6):553-557.

241 Seguin L, Touzani R, Bouhnik AD, et al. Deterioration of Sexual Health in Cancer Survivors Five Years after Diagnosis: Data from the French National Prospective VICAN Survey. Cancers (Basel). 2020 Nov 20;12(11):3453.

242 Sopfe J, Pettigrew J, Afghahi A, Appiah LC, Coons HL. Interventions to Improve Sexual Health in Women Living with and Surviving Cancer: Review and Recommendations. Cancers (Basel). 2021 Jun 24;13(13):3153.

243 https://www.psychologytoday.com/us/blog/homo-consumericus/201201/use-vibrators-among-american-women. Accessed 6/15/22.

244 Rubin ES, Deshpande NA, Vasquez PJ, Kellogg Spadt S. A Clinical Reference Guide on Sexual Devices for Obstetrician-Gynecologists. Obstet Gynecol. 2019 Jun;133(6):1259-1268.

Lymphedema

245 Vincent S. Paramanandam, et al. Prophylactic Use of Compression Sleeves Reduces the Incidence of Arm Swelling in Women at High Risk of Breast Cancer–Related Lymphedema: A Randomized Controlled Trial. Journal of Clinical Oncology. Feb 22, 2022.

246 Kasawara KT, Mapa JMR, Ferreira V, et al. Effects of Kinesio Taping on breast cancer-related lymphedema: A meta-analysis in clinical trials. Physiother Theory Pract. 2018 May;34(5):337-345.

247 YOGA Loudon A, Barnett T, Williams A. Yoga, breast cancer-related lymphoedema and well-being: A descriptive report of women's participation in a clinical trial. J Clin Nurs. 2017 Dec;26(23-24):4685-4695.

248 Nelson NL. Breast Cancer-Related Lymphedema and Resistance Exercise: A Systematic Review. J Strength Cond Res. 2016 Sep;30(9):2656-65.

249 Chiu TW, Kong SL, Cheng KF, Leung PC. Treatment of Post-mastectomy Lymphedema with Herbal Medicine: An Innovative Pilot Study. Plast Reconstr Surg Glob Open. 2020 Jun 24;8(6):e2915.

250 Bruns F, Micke O, Bremer M. Current status of selenium and other treatments for secondary lymphedema. J Support Oncol. 2003 Jul-Aug;1(2):121-30.

251 Petrassi C, Mastromarino A, Spartera C. Pycnogenol in chronic venous insufficiency. Phytomedicine. 2000 Oct;7(5):383-8.

252 Yao C, Xu Y, Chen L, et al. Effects of warm acupuncture on breast cancer-related chronic lymphedema: a randomized controlled trial. Curr Oncol. 2016 Feb;23(1):e27-34.

253 Kilmartin L, Denham T, Fu MR, et al. Complementary low-level laser therapy for breast cancer-related lymphedema: a pilot, double-blind, randomized, placebo-controlled study. Lasers Med Sci. 2020 Feb;35(1):95-105.

254 Shaw C, Mortimer P, Judd PA. A randomized controlled trial of weight reduction as a treatment for breast cancer-related lymphedema. Cancer. 2007;110(8):1868-1874.

255 Showalter SL, Brown JC, Cheville AL, Fisher CS, Sataloff D, Schmitz KH. Lifestyle risk factors associated with arm swelling among women with breast cancer. Ann Surg Oncol. 2013 Mar;20(3):842-9.

256 Ali KM, El Gammal ER, Eladl HM. Effect of Aqua Therapy Exercises on Postmastectomy Lymphedema: A Prospective Randomized Controlled Trial. Ann Rehabil Med. 2021 Apr;45(2):131-140.

257 Mooventhan A, Nivethitha L. Scientific evidence- based effects of hydrotherapy on various systems of the body. North Am J Med, Sci 2014 6:199-209.

258 Remien K, Vilella RC. Osteopathic Manipulative Treatment: Lymphatic Procedures. [Updated 2021 Jul 6]. In: StatPearls [Internet]. Treasure Island (FL): StatPearls Publishing; 2021 Jan.

Peripheral Neuropathy

259 Dimitrova A, Murchison C, Oken B. Acupuncture for the Treatment of Peripheral Neuropathy: A Systematic Review and Meta-Analysis. J Altern Complement Med. 2017 Mar;23(3):164-179.

260 Bao T, Zhi I, Baser R, et al. Yoga for Chemotherapy-Induced Peripheral Neuropathy and Fall Risk: A Randomized Controlled Trial. JNCI Cancer Spectr. 2020 Jun 4;4(6):pkaa048.

261 Sommer C, Cruccu G. Topical Treatment of Peripheral Neuropathic Pain: Applying the Evidence. J Pain Symptom Manage. 2017 Mar;53(3):614-629.

262   Di Stefano G, Di Lionardo A, Galosi E, Truini A, Cruccu G. Acetyl-L-carnitine in painful peripheral neuropathy: a systematic review. J Pain Res. 2019 Apr 26;12:1341-1351.

263   Chen J, Shan H, Yang W, Zhang J, Dai H, Ye Z. Vitamin E for the Prevention of Chemotherapy-Induced Peripheral Neuropathy: A meta-Analysis. Front Pharmacol. 2021 May 13;12:684550.

264   Baute V, Zelnik D, Curtis J, Sadeghifar F. Complementary and Alternative Medicine for Painful Peripheral Neuropathy. Curr Treat Options Neurol. 2019 Sep 2;21(9):44.

265   Ibid.

266   Zhang AC, De Silva MEH, MacIsaac RJ, et al. Omega-3 polyunsaturated fatty acid oral supplements for improving peripheral nerve health: a systematic review and meta-analysis. *Nutr Rev.* 2020 Apr 1;78(4):323-341.

267   Lee G, Kim SK. Therapeutic Effects of Phytochemicals and Medicinal Herbs on Chemotherapy-Induced Peripheral Neuropathy. *Molecules.* 2016; 21(9):1252.

268   Li MJ, Liu LY, Chen L, Cai J, Wan Y, Xing GG. Chronic stress exacerbates neuropathic pain via the integration of stress-affect-related information with nociceptive information in the central nucleus of the amygdala. *Pain.* 2017 Apr;158(4):717-739.

Chronic Pain

269   Bacchi S, Palumbo P, Sponta A, Coppolino MF. Clinical pharmacology of non-steroidal anti-inflammatory drugs: a review. *Antiinflamm Antiallergy Agents Med Chem.* 2012;11(1):52-64.

270   Dragan S, Şerban MC, Damian G,et al. Dietary Patterns and Interventions to Alleviate Chronic Pain. *Nutrients.* 2020 Aug 19;12(9):2510.

271   Pagliai G, Giangrandi I, Dinu M, Sofi F, Colombini B. Nutritional Interventions in the Management of Fibromyalgia Syndrome. *Nutrients.* 2020 Aug 20;12(9):2525.

272   Bannuru RR, Osani MC, Al-Eid F, Wang C. Efficacy of curcumin and Boswellia for knee osteoarthritis: Systematic review and meta-analysis. *Semin Arthritis Rheum.* 2018 Dec;48(3):416-429.

273   Di Cesare Mannelli L, Tenci B, Zanardelli M, et al. Widespread pain reliever profile of a flower extract of Tanacetum parthenium. *Phytomedicine.* 2015 Jul 15;22(7-8):752-8.

274   Rondanelli M, Fossari F, Vecchio V, et al. Clinical trials on pain lowering effect of ginger: A narrative review. *Phytother Res.* 2020 Nov;34(11):2843-2856.

275   Luo Y, Wang CZ, Sawadogo R, Tan T, Yuan CS. Effects of Herbal Medicines on Pain Management. *Am J Chin Med.* 2020;48(1):1-16.

276   Geneen LJ, Moore RA, Clarke C, Martin D, Colvin LA, Smith BH. Physical activity and exercise for chronic pain in adults: an overview of Cochrane Reviews. *Cochrane Database Syst Rev.* 2017 Apr 24;4(4):CD011279.

277   Vickers AJ, Vertosick EA, Lewith G, et al. Acupuncture Trialists' Collaboration. Acupuncture for Chronic Pain: Update of an Individual Patient Data Meta-Analysis. *J Pain.* 2018 May;19(5):455-474.

278   Witt CM, Lüdtke R, Baur R, Willich SN. Homeopathic treatment of patients with chronic low back pain: A prospective observational study with 2 years' follow-up. *Clin J Pain.* 2009 May;25(4):334-9.

279   Bae G, Kim S, Lee S, Lee WY, Lim Y. Prolotherapy for the patients with chronic musculoskeletal pain: systematic review and meta-analysis. *Anesth Pain Med* (Seoul). 2021 Jan;16(1):81-95.

280   Deng G. Integrative Medicine Therapies for Pain Management in Cancer Patients. *Cancer J.* 2019 Sep/Oct;25(5):343-348.

281   Ibid.

Susceptibility to Viral and Other Infections

282   Lova Sun, MD, Sanjna Surya, BS, Anh N Le, BS, et al. Rates of COVID-19–Related Outcomes in Cancer Compared With Noncancer Patients. *JNCI Cancer Spectrum*, Volume 5, Issue 1, February 2021, pkaa120.

283   2 Singh AK, Gupta R, Ghosh A, Misra A. Diabetes in COVID-19: Prevalence, pathophysiology, prognosis and practical considerations. *Diabetes Metab Syndr.* 2020 Jul-Aug;14(4):303-310.

284   Bradley R, Sherman KJ, Catz S, Calabrese C, Oberg EB, Jordan L, Grothaus L, Cherkin DC. Adjunctive naturopathic care for type 2 diabetes: Patient-reported and clinical outcomes after one year. *BMC Complementary and Alternative Medicine.* 2012. 12:44.

285   Meltzer DO, Best TJ, Zhang H, Vokes T, Arora V, Solway J. Association of Vitamin D Deficiency and Treatment with COVID-19 Incidence. *medRxiv [Preprint].* 2020 May 13:2020.05.08.20095893.

286   Lise Alschuler, L., Weil, Andrew, Horwitz,R. et al. Integrative considerations during the COVID-19 pandemic. *Explore.* Volume 16, Issue 6, November–December 2020, Pages 354-356.

287   Skalny AV, Rink L, Ajsuvakova OP, Aschner M, et al. Zinc and respiratory tract infections: Perspectives for COVID19 (Review). *Int J Mol Med.* 2020 Jul;46(1):17-26.

288   16. Read SA, Obeid S, Ahlenstiel C, Ahlenstiel G. The Role of Zinc in Antiviral Immunity. *Adv Nutr.* 2019 Jul 1;10(4):696-710.

289   Colunga Biancatelli RML, Berrill M, Catravas JD, Marik PE. Quercetin and Vitamin C: An Experimental, Synergistic Therapy for the Prevention and Treatment of SARS-CoV-2 Related Disease (COVID-19). *Front Immunol.* 2020 Jun 19;11:1451.

290   Kim Y, Kim H, Bae S, et al. Vitamin C Is an Essential Factor on the Anti-viral Immune Responses through the Production of Interferon-α/β at the Initial Stage of Influenza A Virus (H3N2) Infection. *Immune Netw.* 2013 Apr;13(2):70-4.

291   Kinoshita E, Hayashi K, Katayama H, Hayashi T, Obata A. Anti-influenza virus effects of elderberry juice and its fractions. *Biosci Biotechnol Biochem.* 2012;76(9):1633-8.

292   Lindequist U, Niedermeyer TH, Jülich WD. The pharmacological potential of mushrooms. *Evid Based Complement Alternat Med.* 2005 Sep;2(3):285-99.

293   Bayan L, Koulivand PH, Gorji A. Garlic: a review of potential therapeutic effects. Avicenna *J Phytomed.* 2014 Jan;4(1):1-14.

294   Borugă O, Jianu C, Mişcă C, Goleţ I, Gruia AT, Horhat FG. Thymus vulgaris essential oil: chemical composition and antimicrobial activity. *J Med Life.* 2014;7 Spec No. 3. 56-60.

295   Miraj S, Rafieian-Kopaei, Kiani S. Melissa officinalis L: A Review Study with an Antioxidant Prospective. *J Evid Based Complementary Altern Med.* 2017 Jul;22(3):385-394.

296   Srinivasan V, Mohamed M, Kato H. Melatonin in bacterial and viral infec-tions with focus on sepsis: a review. *Recent Pat Endocr Metab Immune Drug Discov.* 2012 Jan;6(1):30-9.

297   Kim HR, Oh SK, Lim W, Lee HK, Moon BI, Seoh JY. Immune enhancing ef-fects of Echinacea purpurea root extract by reducing regulatory T cell number and function. *Nat Prod Commun.* 2014 Apr;9(4):511-4.

298   Bode AM, Dong Z. *The Amazing and Mighty Ginger.* Herbal Medicine: Biomolecular and Clinical Aspects. 2nd edition. Boca Raton, Florida. CRC Press/Taylor & Francis; 2011. Chapter 7.

299   Abuelgasim H, Albury C, Lee J. Effectiveness of honey for symptomatic relief in upper respiratory tract infections: a systematic review and meta-analysis. *BMJ Evid Based Med.* 2021 Apr;26(2):57-64.

300   Andersen L, Corazon SSS, Stigsdotter UKK. Nature Exposure and Its Effects on Immune System Functioning: A Systematic Review. *Int J Environ Res Public Health.* 2021 Feb 3;18(4):1416.

301   Fixsen A. Homeopathy in the Age of Antimicrobial Resistance: Is It a Vi-able Treatment for Upper Respiratory Tract Infections? Homeopathy. 2018 May;107(2):99-114.

302   Reiman JM, Das B, Sindberg GM, et al. Humidity as a nonpharmaceutical intervention for influenza A. *PLoS One.* 2018 Sep 25;13(9):e0204337.

303   Stephen A. Martin, Brandt D. Pence, Jeffrey A. Woods. Exercise and Re-spiratory Tract Viral Infections *Exerc Sport Sci Rev.* 2009 October;37(4): 157–164.

304   Perez V, Uddin M, Galea S, Monto AS, Aiello AE. Stress, adherence to preventive measures for reducing influenza transmission and influenza-like illness. *J Epidemiol Community Health.* 2012 Jul;66(7):605-10.

305 Sarkar D, Jung MK, Wang HJ. Alcohol and the Immune System. *Alcohol Res.* 2015;37(2):153–5.

306 Brice Faraut, Thomas Andrillon, Marie-Françoise Vecchierini, Damien Leger, Napping: A public health issue. From epidemiological to laboratory studies, *Sleep Medicine Reviews*, Volume 35, 2017, Pages 85-100.

307 Besedovsky L, Lange T, Haack M. The Sleep-Immune Crosstalk in Health and Disease. *Physiol Rev.* 2019 Jul 1;99(3):1325-1380.

308 Büechi S, Vögelin R, von Eiff M, M, Ramos M, Melzer J: Open Trial to Assess Aspects of Safety and Efficacy of a Combined Herbal Cough Syrup with Ivy and Thyme. *Sch Komplementarmed Klass Naturheilkd* 2005;12:328-332.

Chapter 18: Primary Prevention, Medical Research, Clinical Trials, Therapies on the Horizon, and Hopes for the Future

309 Krstic MN, Mijac DD, Popovic DD, Pavlovic Markovic A, Milosavljević T. General Aspects of Primary Cancer Prevention. *Dig Dis.* 2019;37(5):406-415.

310 The Role of Clinical Trial Participation in Cancer Research: Barriers, Evidence, and Strategies. *Am Soc Clin Oncol Educ Book.* 2016;35:185-98.

311 Randall J. Cohrs, Tyler Martin, Parviz Ghahramani, Luc Bidaut, Paul J. Higgins, Aamir Shahzad. Translational Medicine definition by the European Society for Translational Medicine,2015; Pages 86-88.

312 Hoption Cann SA, van Netten JP, van Netten C. Dr William Coley and tumour regression: a place in history or in the future. Postgrad Med J. 2003 Dec;79(938):672-80. PMID: 14707241; PMCID: PMC1742910.

313 Hurwitz MD, et. al. Hyperthermia combined with radiation for the treatment of locally advanced prostate cancer: long-term results from Dana-Farber Cancer Institute study 94-153. *Cancer.* 2011 Feb 1;117(3):510-6.

314 Skitzki JJ, Repasky EA, Evans SS. Hyperthermia as an immunotherapy strategy for cancer. Curr Opin Investig Drugs. 2009;10(6):550-8.

315 M. Ellegaard, et.al. Interleukin-2-induced fever in relation to objective tumor response and survival in patients with metastatic melanoma. Journal of Clinical Oncology 2010 28:15_suppl, 8569-8569.

316 Böttger F, Vallés-Martí A, Cahn L, Jimenez CR. High-dose intravenous vitamin C, a promising multi-targeting agent in the treatment of cancer. J Exp Clin Cancer Res. 2021 Oct 30;40(1):343.

317 Latte-Naor S, Mao JJ. Putting Integrative Oncology into Practice: Concepts and Approaches. *J Oncol Pract.* 2019 Jan;15(1):7-14.

318 Stussman BJ, Nahin RR, Barnes PM, Ward BW. U.S. Physician Recommendations to Their Patients About the Use of Complementary Health Approaches. *J Altern Complement Med.* 2020 Jan;26(1):25-33.